Practices of Anorectal Surgery

Dong Keun Lee
Editor

Practices of Anorectal Surgery

Springer

Editor
Dong Keun Lee
Hansol Hospital
Seoul
South Korea

ISBN 978-981-13-1446-9 ISBN 978-981-13-1447-6 (eBook)
https://doi.org/10.1007/978-981-13-1447-6

This Springer imprint is published by the registered company Springer Nature Singapore Pte Ltd.
The registered company address is: 152 Beach Road, #21-01/04 Gateway East, Singapore 189721, Singapore

Contents

1 Anorectal Anatomy

Choon Sik Chung

1.1 Introduction

The anorectum is the distal part of the gastrointestinal tract protected by muscles, ligaments, and connective tissues attached to the pelvic bones together with the urogenital systems, and it plays an important role in in the regulation of the storage and passage of the stool. The rectum starting at the rectosigmoid junction is connected to the anus through the pelvic floor. The lower 1/3 of the rectum is located outside the peritoneum and is surrounded by Denonvilliers' fascia (Fig. 1.1). Through endoscopy, the rectum has three distinctive wrinkles, which are called the valves of Houston, with the upper and the lower part bent convexly to the right and the middle part to the left (Fig. 1.2). The middle part is approximately the same height as the height of anterior peritoneal reflection and is about 7 cm from the anal verge. The lower part of the rectum is called the rectal ampulla or inferior rectum as the inner space is wider than the upper rectum [1–3].

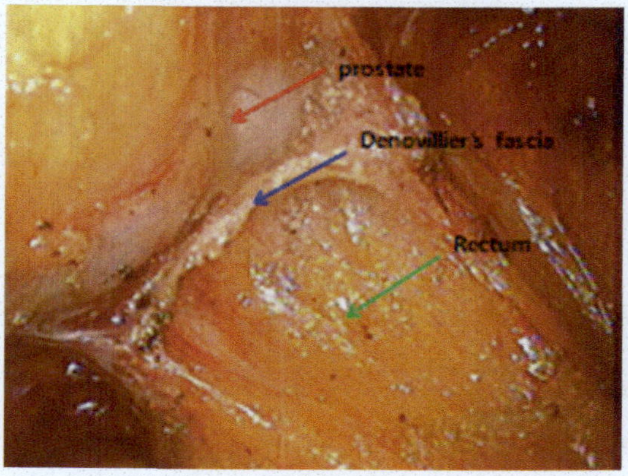

Fig. 1.1 Denonvilliers' fascia (blue line) is a membranous layer at the lowest part of the rectovesical fossa. It separates the prostate and urinary bladder from the rectum. The prostate (red line) and rectum (green line) during laparoscopic anterior resection for rectal cancer

Just like the rectum, a surgeon and an anatomist have different views on the definition of the anal canal [4]. Anatomical definition of the anal canal is from the dentate line to the anal verge. Surgical anal canal is composed of internal and external sphincter muscles and puborectalis muscle, extending from the anal verge to the anorectal ring, and the length is about 4.4 cm in men and 4.0 cm in women, which is the height of the proximal puborectalis muscle [5]. Anorectal ring is a functionally important muscle ring surrounding the junction of the rectum and the anus, composed of the upper side of the anal sphincter and the puborectalis muscle. The rectal mucosa becomes narrower and wrinkles as it moves to the

C. S. Chung (✉)
Colorectal Division, Department of Surgery,
Hansol Hospital, Seoul, South Korea

D. K. Lee (ed.), *Practices of Anorectal Surgery*, https://doi.org/10.1007/978-981-13-1447-6_1

anus, and this is called column of Morgagni, and in the base, it forms a pocket which is called an anal valve. As aligned anal valves look similar to teeth, it is called the dentate line. The dentate line is located approximately 2 cm proximal from the anal verge and about middle of the internal sphincter [6]. The origin of the dentate line is the junction point of the endoderm and ectoderm. Transitional zone around the dentate line differs in the histological structure, innervation, vascular supply, and lymphatic drainage from the rectal mucosa [7]. The anal valve, which is the base of the anal columns, connects to the anal gland via the anal duct through the internal anal sphincter. Around four to eight anal glands concentrated on the posterior side of the anus between the sphincter muscles drained into the anal crypt along with the anal duct (Fig. 1.3) [1, 6].

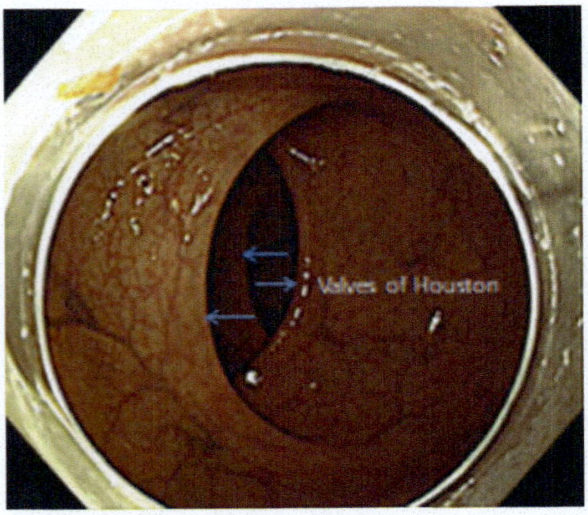

Fig. 1.2 The valves of Houston in the colonoscopic view in the lower rectum. The upper and the lower part bent convexly to the right and the middle part to the left

The anal mucosa of 1~1.5 cm distal to the dentate line is composed of dermal squamous epithelium. The anorectal mucosa is composed of three different epithelial cells depending on the location. The mucosa 1 cm above the dentate line is composed of columnar epithelium like the rectum and progressively migrates to the transition epithelium and the skin-like epithelium [8, 9]. The anal mucosa located between the dentate line and the anal verge is composed of a middle-layer squamous epithelium without any skin appendages such as hair follicles or other skin appendages. The skin in the outside of the anus has radial wrinkles around the anus. The skin of the anal verge is thicker and more pigmented and has hair follicles, sebaceous glands, sweat glands, and apocrine glands and transited to a keratinized stratified squamous epithelium, in other words, to a normal skin (Fig. 1.2) [10].

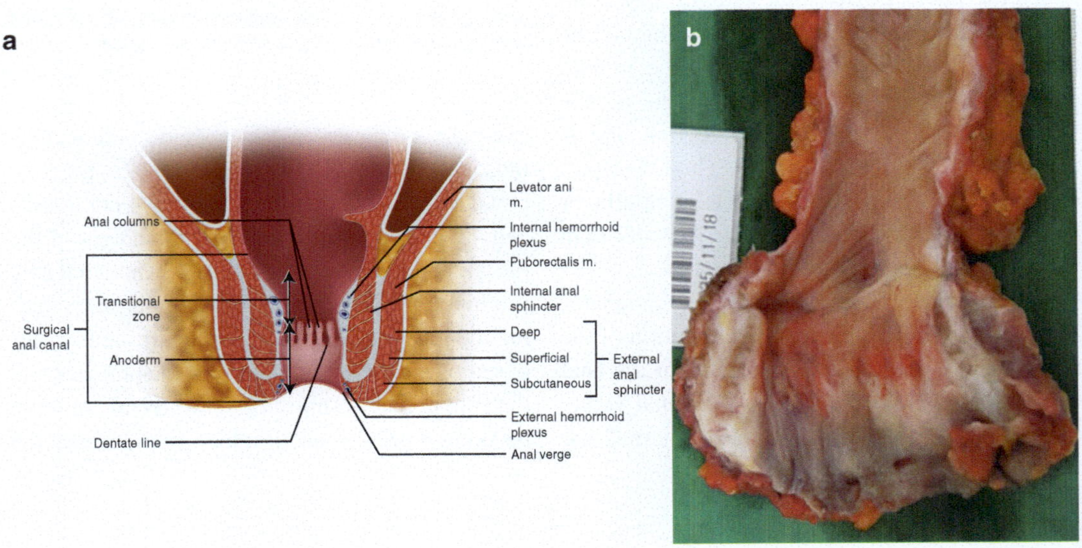

Fig. 1.3 (**a**) Surgical anal canal is composed of internal and external sphincter muscles and puborectalis muscle, extending from the anal verge to the anorectal ring. (**b**) Resected specimen of the anorectum shows the dentate line 2 cm proximal to the anal verge

1.2 Muscular System

The pelvic muscles can be classified into three categories: (1) muscles attached along the pelvic bones, (2) pelvic floor muscles, and (3) anal sphincter muscles.

1.2.1 Pelvic Floor Muscles

The obturator internus and piriformis muscles form the outer boundary of the pelvis, which is not significant in terms of anorectal disease; however, it can be the pathway for infection. Infection from the cryptoglandular complex to deep postanal space can be the pathway for spread of infection to the ischiorectal or ischioanal space.

The pelvic floor (pelvic diaphragm) is a funnel-shaped muscular tendon innervated by S3–S4 and supports organs in peritoneal and pelvic cavities and passes the anorectum and urogenital tract through the hiatus [11]. The pelvic floor muscles originate from the continuous arcus tendineus of the obturator fascia and are symmetric structure of the left and right, the central axis of the pelvis consisting of the iliococcygeus, pubococcygeus, and puborectalis (Fig. 1.4) [12].

The puborectalis muscle is located at the innermost side of the pelvic floor muscle and is located above the deep external sphincter. It's a strong unstriated muscle in U-shaped ring structure forming the anorectal angle at the anorectal junction by pulling the anorectal junction to the posterior pubis. Like the external sphincter, it is

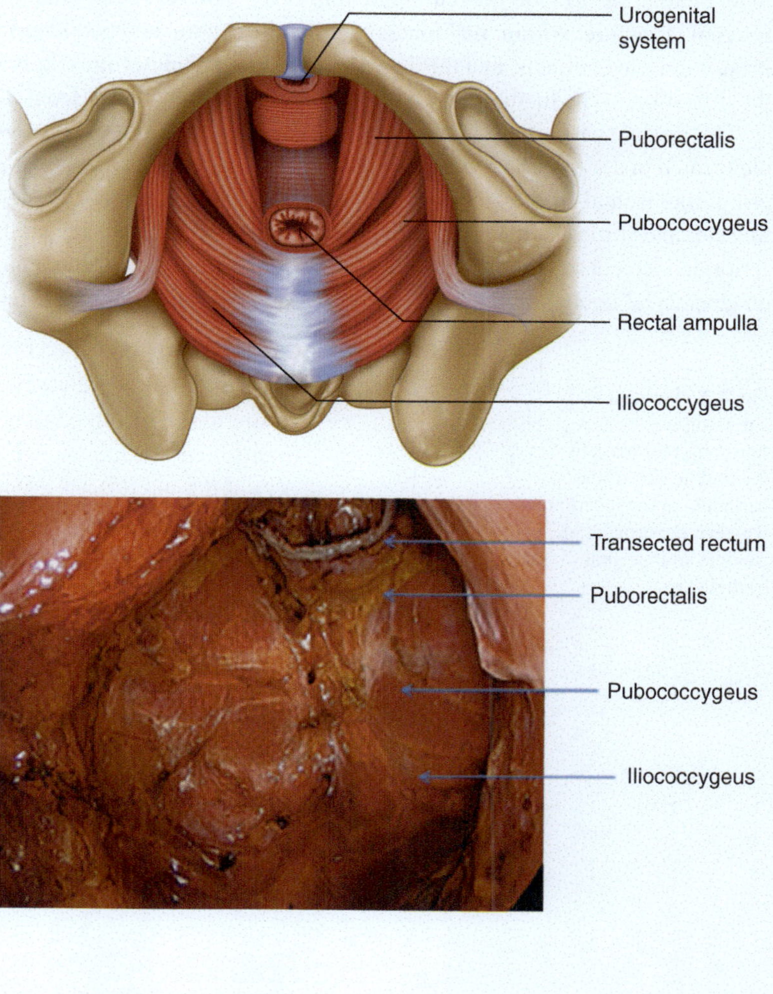

Fig. 1.4 Pelvic floor muscle. Laparoscopic view of the pelvic floor following resection of the rectum

innervated by the inferior rectal nerve of the pudendal nerve [13]. In front of the pelvis, through the hiatus between the two strands from the puborectalis, the rectum, vagina, urethra, and dorsal vein of the penis pass through the pelvic floor. The puborectalis ring relaxes during bowel movement and widens the anorectal angle and straightens the rectum to facilitate defecation. Pelvic floor muscles contract and pull up the pelvic floor at rest [7].

The pubococcygeus muscle is located in the anterior half of the obturator fascia and in the posterior aspect of the pubic bone. It runs in the anterior and posterior direction and engages with the opposite side, which is called the anococcygeal raphae or anococcygeal ligament, and forms the levator hiatus. In birth injury, the pubococcygeus muscle is mainly injured and is a major cause of female pelvic organ prolapse [11]. Fibers of the anococcygeal ligament are arranged in an alternating array to prevent tightening of an internal structure within the hiatus, while the levator muscle contracts, and this has an effect on the dilatation of the hiatus.

The iliococcygeus muscle is a very thin muscle located in the posterior endopelvic fascia covering the ischial spine and internal obturator muscle, and it runs to the interior and posteroinferior and attaches to the lateral of the S4–S5 and anococcygeal ligament.

1.2.2 Perineal Body

The perineal body located in front of the anus supports the perineal region tendinous intersection like the muscular tendon with superficial and deep transverse perineal muscles, and part of the muscle fibers from external sphincter muscles and bulbocavernosus separates the anus from the vagina (Fig. 1.5) [14–16]. Therefore, sphincter injury surgery should restore not only the sphincter but also the perineal body.

1.2.3 Anal Sphincter Muscles

The internal and external sphincter muscles of the anus are a one unit, but their function and structure are quite different. An internal sphincter muscle is a smooth muscle and a continuous muscle of an inner longitudinal muscle of the rectum, and its length is 2.5–4 cm. The internal sphincter muscle is innervated by an autonomic sympathetic from L5 and the parasympathetic nerve from S2 to S4 and has a hypoechoic ring with a thickness of 2–3 mm on the anal ultrasonography [17]. The internal sphincter muscle is responsible for 50–85% of resting anal pressure and closes the anus at resting time [18, 19]. Conversely, the external sphincter muscle is com-

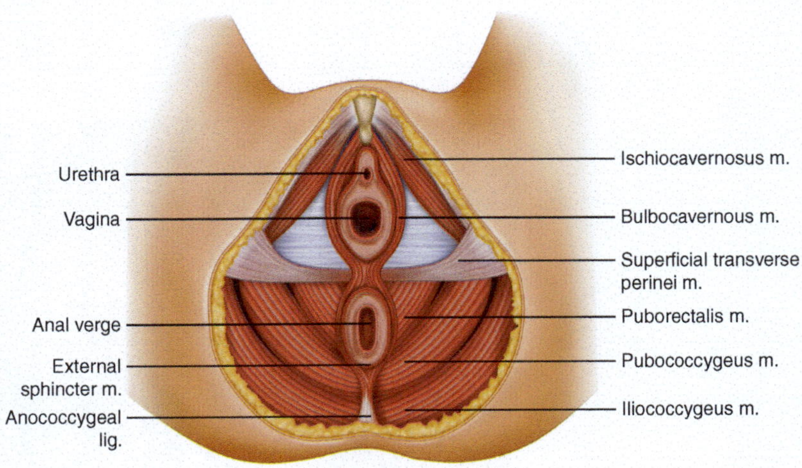

Fig. 1.5 Perineal body, a pyramidal fibromuscular mass in the middle line of the perineum at the junction between the urogenital triangle and the anal triangle

posed of striated muscle and is innervated by the inferior rectal branch of the pudendal nerve. The internal sphincter muscle is terminated at about 1 cm proximal distal of the external sphincter muscle, looking as it is wrapped with the external sphincter muscle, and it is called intersphincteric groove as it is slightly dented under the digital examination. The external sphincter muscle is divided into deep, superficial, and subcutaneous external sphincter, but surgical significance is not great, and it is now considered as a continuous sheet of the skeletal muscle. At the level of the anorectal junction, the deep part of the external sphincter muscle is continued with the puborectalis, and the middle part of the external sphincter muscle runs posterior and attaches to the posterior side of the coccyx. In the anterior side, it forms a perineal body with transverse perineal muscle. The length of the anterior side of the external sphincter muscle in the female is shorter than those of the male on the ultrasonography and MRI [9, 20, 21].

The conjoined longitudinal muscle is formed together with an outer longitudinal muscle of the rectum and striated muscle of the levator muscle at the anorectal ring and descends between the sphincter muscles and passes through the subcutaneous external sphincter muscle to form the corrugator cutis ani (Fig. 1.6) [22, 23]. In some cases, this structure affects hemorrhoids and anal prolapse due to a shearing force generated during defecation and degeneration caused by aging. And also due to the net effect of this muscle, it is functionally less affected even with sphincter injury during hemorrhoidectomy [24]. These muscles also branch off from the sphincter area and compartmentalize nearby tissues to prevent spread of local infections or thrombosis. Some

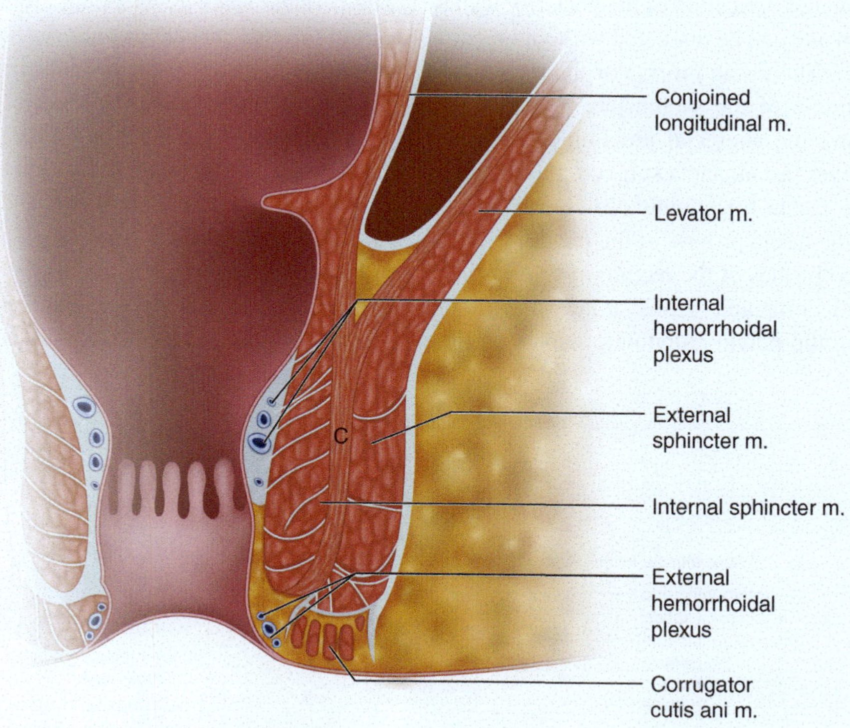

Fig. 1.6 Relationship of the hemorrhoidal plexus with the conjoined longitudinal muscle. Muscular fibers based in the conjoined longitudinal muscle and internal sphincter and attach the cushion to the internal sphincter. The cushion is dilatated with blood when defecating and protects the internal sphincter

muscle fibers attach directly on the inferior anal valve across from the internal sphincter, and it is called mucosal suspensory ligament, and others form the diaphragm across the ischioanal fossa and the external sphincter [25].

1.3 Fascia Structures

The fascia structure is an anatomically important surgical index as it is a surgical resection plane and also a pathway of disease such as an abscess. The pelvis is surrounded by an endopelvic fascia composed of two layers of visceral and parietal peritoneum, and the visceral peritoneum keeps the mesorectum intact with a thin, transparent membrane. A space between the visceral and parietal peritoneum is called Holy Plane [26], and when excised in sacral promontory, it has loose areolar tissue without blood vessels between the two layers (retrorectal space) which are the plane of dissection of the posterior wall of the rectum and can be dissected without bleeding [4, 27–29]. The fascia propria of the rectum and anterior fascia of the sacrum are joined at 3 ~ 5 cm above the anorectal junction and become the Waldeyer fascia, and a surgeon must descend below the fascia for complete dissection of the rectum. The fascia propria of the rectum is thickened on both sides of the rectum in anterior peritoneal reflection and forms a lateral ligament containing the pelvic autonomic nerves and the middle rectal artery to attach the rectum to the pelvic sidewall [30]. The rectum is divided laterally from the lateral pelvic wall by the hypogastric nerve, pelvic plexus, and hypogastric artery. Anteriorly Denonvilliers' fascia is formed by the fusion of two peritoneal membranes and divided the rectum from the prostate and seminal vesicles in the male and vagina in the female [1, 31].

1.4 Anorectal Spaces

The lower rectum and perianal tissue are divided into several spaces by the levator muscle and anal sphincter, which is an important anatomical structure for the treatment of abscess and spread of inflammation (Fig. 1.7) [32].

1.4.1 Perianal Space

The perianal space is wrapping around the distal part of the anal canal and continues laterally to the subcutaneous fat of buttocks. In the perianal space, an external hemorrhoidal plexus communicates with the upper internal hemorrhoidal plexus at the dentate line. The perianal space is the lowest part of the external and internal sphincter and has the corrugator cutis ani muscle fiber which acts as a kind of lattice to have thrombus or abscess to remain in the restricted area; therefore, pain becomes rather severe with sudden increase of pressure.

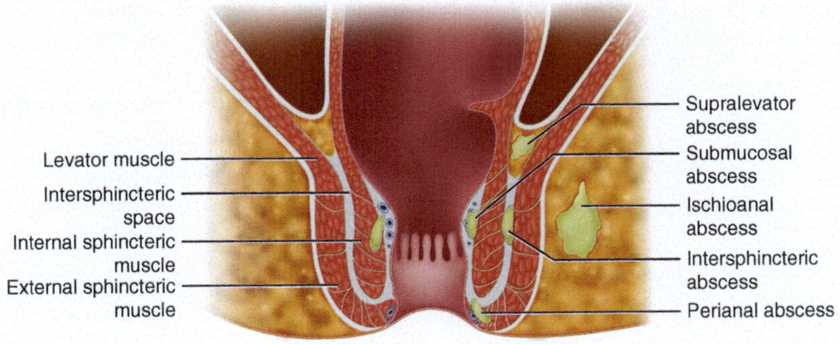

Fig. 1.7 Anorectal spaces are comprised of the levator muscle and the anal sphincter including the ischiorectal, perianal, intersphincteric, submucous, superficial and deep postanal, supralevator, and retrorectal space

1.4.2 Submucosal Space

In the dentate line, there is an internal hemorrhoidal plexus and a muscularis mucosa in the space between the internal sphincter and submucosal layer of the distal rectum just above the dentate line.

1.4.3 Intersphincteric Space

The intersphincteric space is located between the internal and external sphincter muscles and has the anal gland and connects downward to the perianal space. Most of the perianal inflammation begins and spreads through this area [19].

1.4.4 Ischiorectal/Ischioanal Space

The ischioanal space is the largest of the perianal space and is, however, distinguished from the other perianal spaces by the fascia of the levator muscle on the upper side, the external sphincter on the medial side, the obturator fascia on the lateral side, and the thin transverse fascia on the lower side, and aside from fat tissue, it also has the pudendal nerve which comes out of Alcock's canal and the medial pudendal artery. In the posterior side of the anus, the superficial and Courtney's deep postanal space are connected to the ischioanal space from both sides, which is the passage for the formation of horseshoe abscess [33].

1.4.5 Superficial and Deep Postanal Space

The superficial postanal space is located between the skin and the anococcygeal ligament, and the deep rectosphincteric space of Courtney is located between the anococcygeal ligament and the anococcygeal raphae.

1.4.6 Supralevator Space

The levator muscle located between the pelvic and peritoneal cavity divides the pelvis into the supralevator space and the infralevator space. The supralevator space communicates with the ischiorectal space through the internal fascia of the obturator muscle, where the supralevator abscess passes to the perianal space.

1.5 Anorectal Vascular System

1.5.1 Arterial Blood Supply

The rectum is supplied by the median sacral artery and upper, middle, and lower rectal artery. The upper rectal artery is the terminal branch of the inferior mesenteric artery and is characterized by a network formation by communication with the middle rectal artery in the submucosa of the rectum (Fig. 1.8) [34].

The middle rectal artery originates from the internal iliac artery or inferior vesicle artery and surrounds the nervi erigentes along the pelvic sidewall and feeds blood to both sides of the rectum from the upper side to the middle of the pelvic floor muscle. And in 25% of the cases, it is present only in one side [35]. The lower rectum and anus have blood supply from the superior rectal artery and the inferior hemorrhoidal artery, and some are supplied from the middle rectal artery, forming a rich submucosal intersecting network [36, 37]. The pudendal artery from the internal iliac artery together with the pudendal nerve from Alcock's canal branches off to the inferior hemorrhoidal artery. The median sacral artery is located in the posterior portion of the abdominal aortic branch, descends posterior to the rectum, branches to the rectum from the end of the coccyx, and may cause bleeding during anterior or low anterior resection.

1.5.2 Venous Drainage

The rectal vein runs the same anatomically with the artery. The venous blood of the lower rectum and anus is collected in the arteriovenous plexus and enters the vena cava through the internal iliac vein through the middle/lower hemorrhoidal vein. External hemorrhoidal plexus is located in the perianal fossa below the dentate line, and the internal hemorrhoidal plexus is in the upper submucosal layer and communicates with each other (Fig. 1.9) [32, 38].

1.6 Innervation of the Anorectum

The colon and rectum are innervated by sympathetic and parasympathetic nerves, and the external anal sphincter muscle and anal mucosa are innervated by the somatic nerve. The parasympathetic nerve (autonomic nervous system of the brain) increases peristalsis and secretory activity and relaxes the ileocecal valve and sphincter muscles. The sympathetic nerves (T12–L2) work in opposition to parasympathetic nerves. The dis-

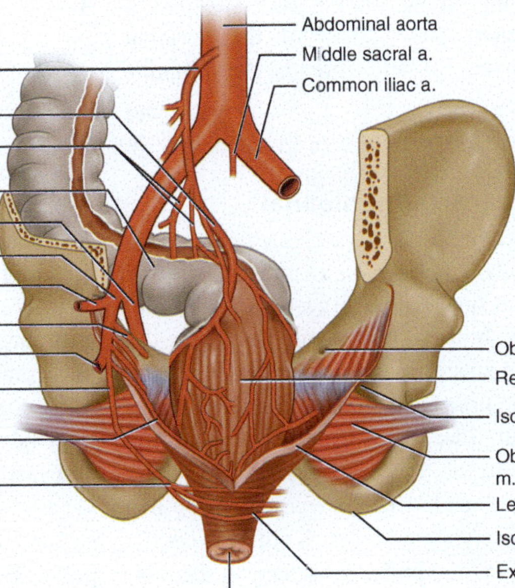

Fig. 1.8 Arterial supply of the pelvic floor and the rectum. The rectum is mainly supplied by the superior rectal artery arising as a main branch of the inferior mesenteric artery

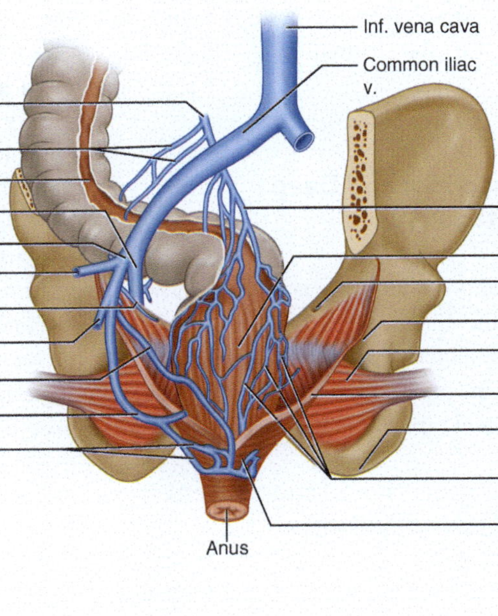

Fig. 1.9 Venous drainage of the pelvic floor and the rectum. The venous drainage of the rectum is to the inferior mesenteric vein into the portal system

tribution of the autonomic nervous system travels close to the artery. The autonomic nervous system of the pelvic rectum is composed of two important neural dominances: hypogastric nerve and pelvic neural complex [25, 26]. In the thoracolumbar sympathetic ganglia, postganglionic fibers descend along the posterior peritoneum just before the abdominal aorta and are called the inferior mesenteric nerve at the aortic site near the mesenteric artery and two inferior mesenteric nerves at the abdominal aorta. It is branched to the lower nerve and branches into two hypogastric nerves at the aortic bifurcation. The inferior mesenteric nerve and the hypogastric nerve can be easily identified by opening the peritoneum in the anterior sacrum, and they can be easily traced with the inferior mesenteric artery. Therefore, care should be taken not to damage these nerves when cutting the lower mesenteric artery or superior rectal artery [31]. Each hypogastric nerve descends along with the posterior wall of the rectum and combines with the nervi erigentes of the pelvic sidewall to form the pelvic plexus, which controls the prostate, seminal vesicle, and urethra anterolaterally. The visceral preganglionic fibers form the plexus, which is known as nervi erigentes, coming out from the bilateral sacral foramens (S2, S3, S4) [38]. Each pelvic plexus is located at the origin of the middle rectal artery. The pelvic nerve meets the hypogastric nerves and makes pelvic plexus, which innervates the rectum, bladder, seminal vesicle, and urethra. Ejaculation depends on the input of the sympathetic nerves of the pelvic plexus and the pelvic nerves. The true hindgut is ultimately innervated by parasympathetic nerves of the thoracic lumbar plexus in a retrograde form of the pelvic nerve, plexus, and hypogastric nerve. The pudendal nerves originating from S2 to S4 pass through Alcock's canal formed by the medial fascia of the internal obturator muscle and travel to the external pelvis to the ischiorectal pouch and ramifies to the lower rectal artery, perineal nerve, and dorsal nerve of the penis and clitoris (Fig. 1.10). The motor innervation of the upper side of the pelvic floor muscle is innervated by S2–S4, and the lower side is innervated by the perineal branch of the pudendal nerve [28]. The puborectalis is innervated by the inferior rectal nerve and the external sphincter by the lower rectal branch of the pudendal nerve (S2, S3) and the perineal branch of S4. The internal sphincter muscle is a continuous muscle of the rectal smooth muscle; it is innervated by sympathetic (L5) and parasympathetic (S2–S4) nerves like the rectum. The sensory nerve of the anal canal is the borderline about 0.3 ~ 1.5 cm from the dentate line. The rectum above this borderline is transferred to the parasympathetic nerve and afferent fibers of the pelvic nerve plexus with only the sense of dilatation to S2–S4. An anal sensory is considered to play an important role in

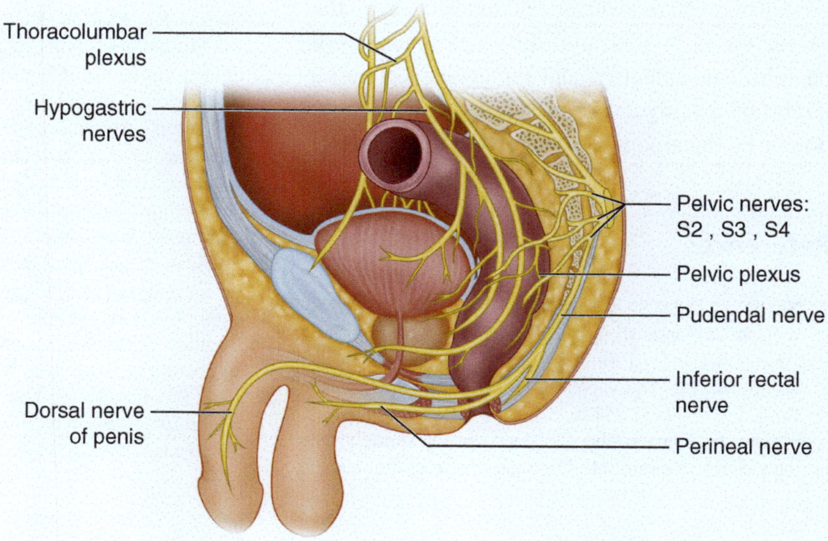

Fig. 1.10 Innervation of the anorectum. The rectum is innervated by sympathetic and parasympathetic nerves, and the external anal sphincter muscle and anal mucosa are innervated by the somatic nerve

the bowel control and has a sense of touch, pinprick, heat, and cold. They are innervated by the lower rectal branch of the pudendal nerve.

1.7 Lymphatic Drainage

Lymphatic drainage of the rectum is parallel to the running of arterial blood. In rectal cancer, most of metastatic lymph nodes are found in the posterior mesorectum of the upper 2/3 of the rectum [39, 40].

Abundant lymphatic plexus in the anus and rectum is drained into extramural lymph nodes and lymphatic plexus. The dentate line is located between the other two lymphatic systems, draining into the inferior mesenteric and internal iliac lymph nodes at the upper portion and superficial inguinal lymph nodes at the 1/3 of the lower portion. The upper 2/3 of the rectum is drained into the inferior mesenteric lymph node and the para-aortic lymph node, and the lower 1/3 of the rectum is drained into superior rectum and inferior mesenteric lymph nodes, and the others are drained into the internal iliac lymph node along the middle rectal artery [41].

1.8 Summary

Prior to the treatment, an accurate clinical and physical diagnosis is necessary. Especially anal sphincter is a key factor in the bowel control, and it is difficult to recover once damaged. Also, the anorectum is divided into different zones based on sphincter anatomy, and the zones can be an important passage for the spread of inflammation or be the area where the abscesses stagnate.

References

1. Shafik A, Doss S, Ali YA, et al. Transverse folds of rectum: anatomic study and clinical implications. Clin Anat. 2001;14(3):196–203.
2. Abramson DJ. The valves of Houston in adults. Am J Surg. 1978;136(3):334–6.
3. Saleno G, Sinnatamby C, Branagan G, Daniels IR, Heald RJ, Moran BJ. Defining the rectum: surgically, radiologically and anatomically. Colorectal Dis. 2006;8(Suppl 3):5–9.
4. Wendell-Smith CP. Anorectal nomenclature: fundamental terminology. Dis Colon Rectum. 2000;43:1349–58. P.1-26.
5. Nivatvongs S, Stern HS, Fryd DS. The length of the anal canal. Dis Colon Rectum. 1981;24:600–1.
6. Klosterhalfen B, Offner F, Vogel P, et al. Anatomic nature and surgical significance of anal sinus and anal intramuscular glands. Dis Colon Rectum. 1991;34:156–60.
7. Heald RJ, Moran BJ. Embryology and anatomy of the rectum. Semin Surg Oncol. 1998;15(2):66–71.
8. Fenger C. The anal transitional zone. Acta Pathol Microbiol Immunol Scand Suppl. 1987;289(supplement):1–42.
9. Fenger C. The anal canal epithelium. A review. Scand J Gastroenterol Suppl. 1979;54:114–7.
10. von Seebach HB, Stumm D, Misch P, et al. Hidrocystoma and adenoma of apocrine anal glands. Virchows Arch A Pathol Anat Histol. 1980;386:231–7.
11. Strohbehn K. Normal pelvic floor anatomy. Obstet Gynecol Clin North Am. 1988;25:683–705.
12. Stoker J. Anorectal and pelvic anatomy. Best Pract Rec Clin Gastroenterol. 2009;23:463–75.
13. Fucini C, Elbetti C, Messerini L. Anatomic plane of separation between external anal sphincter and puborectalis muscle: clinical implications. Dis Colon Rectum. 1999;42:374–9.
14. Shafik A. Physioanatomic entirety of external anal sphincter with bulbocavernosus muscle. Arch Androl. 1999;42:45–54.
15. Larson KA, Yousuf A, Lewicky-Gaupp C, Fenner DE, DeLancey JO. Perineal body anatomy I living women: 3-dimensional analysis using thin-slice magnetic resonance imaging. Am J Obstet Gynecol. 2010;203:494.e15–21.
16. Mittal RK, et al. Purse-string morphology of external anal sphincter revealed by novel imaging technique. Am J Physiol Gastrointest Liver Physiol. 2014;306(6):G505–14.
17. Rociu E, Stoker J, Eijkemans MJ, Lame'ris JS. Normal anal sphincter anatomy and age- and sex-related variations at high-spatial resolution endoanal MR imaging. Radiology. 2000;217:395–401.
18. Lawson JO. Structure and function of the internal anal sphincter. Proc R Soc Med. 1970;63:84–9.
19. Gerdes B, Kohler HH, Zielke A, et al. The anatomical basis of anal endosonography. A study in postmortem specimens. Surg Endosc. 1997;11:986–90.
20. Shafic A. A concept of the anatomy of the anal sphincter mechanism and the physiology of defecation. Dis Colon Rectum. 1987;30:970–82.
21. Bogduk N. Issues in anatomy: the external anal sphincter revisited. Aust N Z J Surg. 1996;66:626–9.
22. Haas PA, Fox TA Jr. The importance of the perianal connective tissue in the surgical anatomy and function of the anus. Dis Colon Rectum. 1977;20:303–13.

23. Macchi V, Porzionato A, Stecco C, Vigato E, Parenti A, DeCaro R. Histo-topographic study of the longitudinal anal muscle. Clin Anat. 2008;21:447–52.
24. Thomson WH. The nature of haemorrhoids. Br J Surg. 1975;62:542–52.
25. Lunniss PJ, Phillips RK. Anatomy and function of the anal longitudinal muscle. Br J Surg. 1992;79:882–4.
26. Heald RJ. The 'Holy Plane' of recta surgery. J R Soc Med. 1988;81(9):503–8.
27. Pearl RK, Monsen H, Abcarian H. Surgical anatomy of the pelvic autonomic nerves. A practical approach. Am Surg. 1986;52:236–7.
28. Shafic A, el-Sherif M, Youssef A, et al. Surgical anatomy of the pudendal nerve and its clinical applications. Clin Anat. 1995;8:110–5.
29. Stoss F. Investigation of the muscular architecture of the rectosigmoid junction in humans. Dis Colon Rectum. 1990;33:378–83.
30. Jones OM, Smeulders N, Wiseman O, et al. Lateral ligaments of the rectum: an anatomical study. Br J Surg. 1999;86(4):487–9.
31. Maurer CA. Urinary and sexual function after total mesorectal excision. Recent Results Cancer Res. 2005;165:196–204.
32. Barleben A, Mills S. Anorectal anatomy and physiology. Surg Clin North Am. 2010;90(1):1–15.
33. Llauger J, et al. The normal and pathologic ischiorectal fossa at CT and MR imaging. Radiographics. 1998;18(1):61–82.
34. Schuurman JP, Go PM, Bleys RL. Anatomical branches of the superior rectal artery in the distal rectum. Colorectal Dis. 2009;11(9):967–71.
35. Didio LJ, Diaz-Franco C, Schemainda R, et al. Morphology of the middle rectal arteries: a study of 30 cadaveric dissections. Surg Radiol Anat. 1986;8(4):229–36.
36. Siddharth P, Ravo B. Colorectal neurovasculature and anal sphincter. Surg Clin North Am. 1988;68(6):1185–200.
37. Lund JN, Binch C, McGrath J, et al. topographical distribution of blood supply to the anal canal. Br J Surg. 1999;86:496–8.
38. Sato K, Sato T. The vascular and neuronal composition of the lateral ligament of the rectum and the rectosacral fascia. Surg Radiol Anat. 1991;13:17–22.
39. Wang C, Zhou Z, Wang Z, et al. Patterns of neoplastic foci and lymph node micrometastasis within the mesorectum. Langenbecks Arch Surg. 2005;390(4):312–8.
40. Topor B, Acland R, Kolodko V, et al. Mesorectal lymph nodes: their location and distribution within the mesorectum. Dis Colon Rectum. 2003;46(6):779–85.
41. Canessa CE, Badia F, Fierro S, et al. Anatomic study of the lymph nodes of the mesorectum. Dis Colon Rectum. 2001;44:1333–6.

Anorectum Physiology

2

Yong Geul Joh

2.1 Introduction

The most vital function of the anorectum is the bowel control and continence. A normal bowel control has a complex interaction with rectal sensation, coordination of the anal muscle and pelvic floor muscle, rectal compliance, stool consistency, and innervation. If one or more factors do not work properly, common or rare clinical disease can occur. When referring to an anorectal physiology, it is the information through an examination of various factors provided by the anorectal physiology laboratory. These are the basic tests of anorectal physiology laboratory: resting and squeezing anal pressure, recto-anal inhibitory reflex, dynamic proctography, defecography, rectal compliance, sensory threshold, PNTML, and transanal ultrasonography. However, there have been controversies on the role of laboratory in examining the anorectal abnormalities for a long time, and the utility in the clinic is still not well accepted [1, 2].

2.2 Examination

Prior to selecting the necessary anorectal physiology test, it is important to obtain helpful information from detailed hearing of medical history and after a detailed digital rectal examination (DRE). Be careful to identify the start and duration of the symptom, incidence and consistency of the bowel movement, fiber and fluid intakes, accompanied diseases, and operation history, and also acknowledge the degree of daily activity of the patient. Based on the patient's medical history, it is possible to obtain useful information from physical examination including pelvic examination including digital rectal examination. When performing digital rectal examination, prone kneeling position is the most ideal position; however, considering disconcert of the patient, lateral decubitus position is generally implemented. DRE includes inspection of the perianal and digital examination, and if necessary, anoscopy is also included. Perianal erosion, scar, anal pile, anal fissure, or discharge from the perineum is noticed through the inspection. Also, pinprick test can be identified with light touch of the perianal skin [3]. Digital examination may reveal hemorrhoids, tumor, or the prostate in the anal canal or the rectum and estimate anal pressure of resting and squeezing time. By increasing abdominal pressure, the temporary relaxation of the sphincter muscle can also be checked [4]. The level of accuracy from an experienced doctor's digital examination of anal pressure of resting and squeezing time is about 70% of the anal manometry [5]. But as the physical examination has lower sensitivity and specificity about 50%, various objective evaluation tests are performed to complement these physical examinations [6]. The main clinical focus of anorectal physiology

Y. G. Joh (✉)
Jangnhang Clinic, Hanam, South Korea

D. K. Lee (ed.), *Practices of Anorectal Surgery*, https://doi.org/10.1007/978-981-13-1447-6_2

test is conflicting clinical diseases of constipation and fecal incontinence occurring simultaneously in some cases. Anorectal diseases are often associated with complex pathophysiology, in various forms, especially outlet obstructive constipation, fecal incontinence, and anal pain. Recently, the incidence of these diseases has been increasing with the increase of aging population.

2.3 Basic Anorectal Physiology Laboratory Tests

In order to achieve normal bowel movement, some of anatomical and functional elements should act intimately and complexly. Mechanism of bowel movement starts from the desire to defecate when the rectum is dilated from stool coming into the rectum. At the moment of desire to defecate, the internal sphincter slightly relaxes, and the external sphincter contracts to define whether the content is gas, watery, or solid stool by recto-anal inhibitory reflex. If it is defined as stool, defecation starts in sitting down position in the toilet by increasing the internal rectal pressure and abdominal pressure and relaxing the pelvic muscle, especially the anal sphincter muscle and the puborectalis muscle. Basic anorectal function tests are performed prior to the surgery to give actual help to the clinician in the case with the possibility of dysfunction of bowel movement or with bowel movement disorder. The tests include anorectal manometry, electromyography, dynamic proctography, colon motility test, and anal ultrasonography.

2.3.1 Anal Manometry

The techniques of manometry will not be dealt here. The function of the anal sphincter (resting and contraction period of sphincter pressure), duration of maintaining contraction, measurement of anal sphincter function length, pressure changes from a sudden increase of abdominal pressure like cough, pressure changes during the attempt to defecate, and recto-anal inhibitory reflex can be measured by this test. Resting anal pressure refers to the difference between the anal pressure and the rectal pressure when relaxed and comfortable. The internal sphincter plays a key role of 60–70%, and others; external sphincter 20–30%, anal cushions about 15% for resting pressure [7]. Sphincter length refers to anal canal length which is over 5 mmHg higher in pressure than the internal rectal pressure. Also, high pressure zone refers to the area of anal canal which is higher than the half of maximum resting pressure, and the length is 2.5 ~ 5 cm, and women's length is shorter than that of men [8, 9]. Squeezing anal pressure refers to the difference between the external sphincter pressure and the rectal pressure, which mainly occurs due to the pressure from the external sphincter. During the examination, make sure the patient contracts the anus maximally, and it is important not to contract the other muscles. Contract duration can also be measured; this is the duration of maintaining a pressure higher than the half of maximum squeezing pressure. Like the other anorectal physiology tests, an experienced clinician and equipment are essential, and it takes about 30 minutes for the test. And to achieve a successful result, a laboratory room with an independent and comfortable atmosphere will be needed (Fig. 2.1).

Anorectal manometry is a technique used to measure contractility in the anus and rectum. This technique uses a balloon in the rectum to distend the rectum and a pressure sensor at the internal anal sphincter to measure the presence or absence of the rectosphincteric reflex.

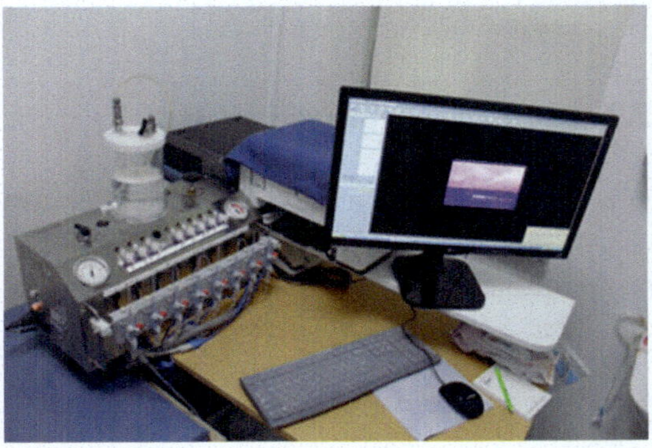

Fig. 2.1 Anorectal manometry

2.3.2 Recto-anal Inhibitory Reflex

In the lower rectum, insert a catheter with a balloon, and inject 50 cc of water or air to make sudden dilatation. In normal cases, the external sphincter contracts followed by relaxing of the internal sphincter, and the resting anal pressure decreases temporarily over 25%. The larger the dilatation of the rectum, the pressure descending is higher, and the duration also lasts longer [10]. This test is a normal process of sampling reflex, which determines the content in the rectum and distinguishes whether to defecate. If this recto-anal inhibitory reflex does not happen, it can be suspected diseases like Hirschsprung or systemic sclerosis. It can be used as a diagnostic tool for chronic constipation and to exclude congenital megacolon, but there are also reports that 10% of the patients without congenital megacolon do not have recto-anal inhibitory reflex. Therefore, the value of using this to an adult constipation cases in clinic is very low [11, 12].

2.3.3 Pudendal Nerve Terminal Motor Latency (PNTML)

PNTML test measures the conduction time of the pudendal nerve from Alcock's canal to the external sphincter. This is to aid patients with pelvic floor dysfunction from neuromuscular disability by evaluating the innervation of the external sphincter. Insert your rubber gloved index finger with latency measuring surface electrode attached into the rectum, and press the left and right ischial spine. Then the contraction of the external sphincter from the index finger can be felt, and measure the time from the point of electric stimulus to the point of maximum amplitude of motor unit reflex [13]. Normal conduction time is 2.0 ± 0.2 msec [14]. A longer conduction time means the damage of large fast-conducting fibers, and the significance of increased conduction time is controversial. The possibility of the sphincter function recovery after the correction surgery from the patients with perineal descent or rectal prolapse caused by constipation can be predicted even though the significance of increased conduction time is controversial. Extended conduction time from the damage of the unilateral pudendal nerve does not affect prognosis of reconstruction surgery of the sphincter muscle; however, functional result of the surgery is poor when the conduction time of both sides has extended [15, 16].

2.3.4 Electromyography (EMG)

Anal electromyography tests are used to determine the function of the sphincter muscles whether it's a neuropathy or a muscular disorder. A functional assessment of pelvic floor activity records the activity of electrical contraction of the puborectalis muscle and the external sphincter muscle during resting, contracting, and defecating period using the anal surface electrode or needle electrode. Needle electrode can measure only the activity unit from the limited muscular fibers; however, it can also cause pain from the needle, and artificial contraction can occur. Surface electrode is convenient with no pain; however, the negative side is that it measures the sum of activity unit from the number of motor units.

Anal surface electrode is wrapped with a small sponge and placed in the anal canal to measure the electrical activity of the pelvic floor muscle including the puborectalis muscle, and the result shows in a recruitment pattern. In other words, when the electrode is placed still, it is the standard activity value; in contraction, the activity increases; and finally when it is straining like bowel movement, it falls below the standard value [17–19]. In the patients with non-relaxing puborectalis, the electrical activity is higher than the activity in the contracting sphincter muscle during bowel movement, which means that the puborectalis contracts rather than relaxes during defecation [20].

2.3.5 Balloon Expulsion Test

This is to simply test defecation ability or holding ability, but it is time-consuming, and therefore it is not easily performed in the clinic. If you combine the tests with other physiological function tests, it is helpful in diagnosing outlet obstructive constipation [21]. Lay your patient on their left, insert balloon-attached catheter into the lower rectum, and inject 50 cc of air or warm water, and make your patient push it out like defecation. A normal person can defecate within 10 seconds. If one can't defecate within 30 seconds, you have to attach the weight on pulley and increase the weight by 100 mg until defecation. And if defecation starts after you put more than 200 mg weight, it can be determined as outlet obstructive constipation [22, 23]. You have to consider that the patient cannot show normal defecation as the examiner is in the room and the anxiety of accidental gas or stool defecation, in that they would not be able to strain enough or relax their anal muscle. Especially, as lying on their left position is not a normal defecation position, this cannot reflect normal bowel habit.

2.3.6 Rectal Compliance Test

In order to hold the defecation, the rectum has to preserve stool coming down through the sigmoid colon for a certain time. But when the rectum is full with stool, receptive relaxation occurs in the rectal wall, and then the rectal internal pressure becomes decreasing prior to dilatation. The dilatation at this status is called rectal compliance. An examination is done to measure the rectal compliance by increasing the pressure of the balloon placed in the rectum by 2 mmHg and calculating the volume pressure from pressure change. Rectal hypersensitivity can be examined in the proctitis patients with absolute change in the compliance due to ulcerative colitis or radiation exposure and also from sporadic diarrhea-dominant irritable bowel syndrome or urgent fecal incontinence.

2.4 Defecography

Defecography and dynamic proctography can examine the process of topodynamic of bowel movement, with the fast changing from the anorectum and pelvic floor during defecation after the injection (contrast medium, isotope, etc.) through the anus, and they are used in identifying pelvic floor function during bowel movement. Video defecography, defecography, and defecating scintigraphy are all the same measurement methods. As for defecography indications, it is when assessing constipation or fecal incontinence, when suspecting rectal prolapse, or in the case of solitary rectal ulcer through endoscope. Mixture of barium and methylcellulose is made similar to stool and placed in the rectum. The patient is sat in a chair, and the examination is carried out to defecate the mixture under fluoroscopic monitoring. By examining the length of anal canal, anorectal border, posterior anorectal angle, central anorectal angle, distance to pubococcygeal line, pubococcygeal line, and the width of anal canal, you can identify the paradoxical contraction in the puborectalis, endorectal intussusception, rectocele, small intestine, perineal descent, and incomplete defecation (Fig. 2.2) [24, 25].

This test may be performed by a triple contrast method. In general angiography, water-soluble barium is administered, and the vagina is filled with dissolved barium. Through this, more accurate anatomical distinction is possible through the rectum, small intestine, and vagina. Sometimes, water-soluble barium is injected directly into abdominal cavity to identify the outline of the pelvis. Rectocele is defined as abnormal findings when protruding more than 3 cm. And perineal descent is defined stable when it's over 4 cm or descends over 3 cm when contracting than stable [26, 27].

2.5 Colon Transit Time

This is a basic method for assessing colon motor function. By measuring the transit time of an entire colon or partial colon, it can help set treatment plan and classify types by pathophysiology in a chronic constipation. Also, it is useful in judging the efficacy after the medical or surgical treatment. As colonic atresia may be accompanied with outlet obstructive constipation, prior to

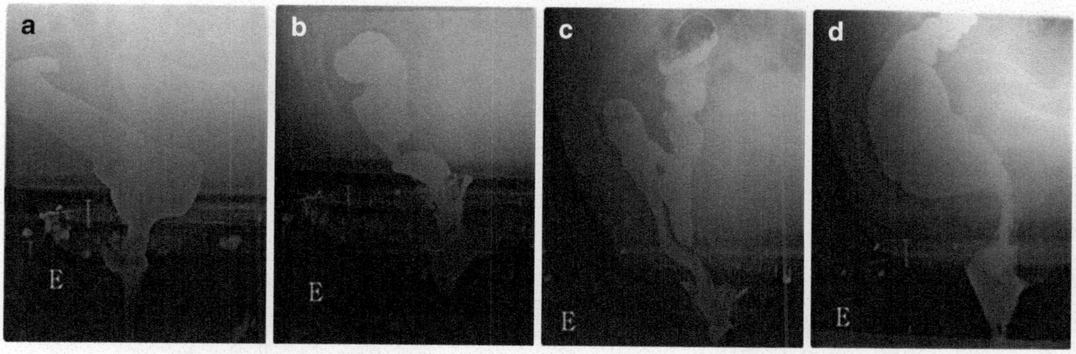

Fig. 2.2 Defecography. (**a**) Rectocele: the anterior rectal wall protrudes over the expected position. (**b**) Rectal intussusception: the prolapsed rectal wall passing through the anal canal and anus during evacuation. (**c**) Rectal prolapse: the anterior rectal wall protrudes into the bulb during evacuation. (**d**) Non-relaxing puborectalis syndrome: abnormally deep puborectal impression at the beginning of the evacuation phase

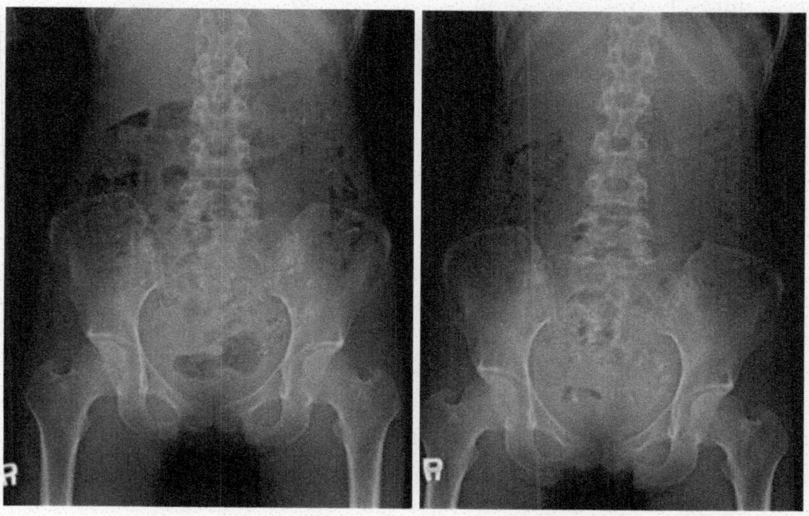

Fig. 2.3 Colon transit time

the surgical treatment of constipation, an examination of colon transit time has to be performed. In a single-marker technique, 20 or 24 radiopaque markers have to be administered in a capsule with water at a scheduled time, and an abdominal tomography is performed on the 3rd, 5th, and 7th days (Fig. 2.3). In multiple-marker techniques, the capsule is administered at a scheduled time for 3 days, and an abdominal X-ray is performed on the 3rd, 5th, 7th, 10th, and 13th days and records the number and distribution of the markers. The transit time calculates the right, left, and rectum sigmoid colon areas and the whole length [28–30].

Twenty radiopaque markers were ingested in the morning, and abdominal X-rays were taken at 24-hr intervals until all markers had been passed. Most healthy, symptom-free subjects passed all markers out of the colon within 4–5 days.

If a marker is scattered all over the colon on the last day of X-ray, it corresponds to the colonic atresia opinion, and if it is gathered in the rectum, it is outlet obstructive constipation. It is recommended to perform an additional examination of outlet obstructive constipation even if it shows an abnormal result of colonic atresia, as it tends to accompany pelvic floor dysfunction.

Differential diagnosis of slow-transit constipation and outlet obstructive constipation can be performed by hearing the medical history, and an examination is performed on the selective patients who are planning to have total colectomy for the slow-transit constipation. But it is difficult for the patient to complete the examination as it takes longer, and for the period, they have to stop the medication. Also, for the assessment, age, gender, and amount of fibrin and fluid intake during the examination have to be considered.

2.6 Transanal Ultrasonography

Anal ultrasonography is the most accurate and complete testing tool for assessing structural abnormalities of an anal sphincter. Generally, a radial transducer with 10 MHz, 360-degree view is used. Through the 3-D imaging ultrasound, it can determine the anal structure by sectional and 3-D (Fig. 2.4). And with having accurate information of sphincter lesion, you can determine rectocele, intussusceptions, cystocele, and sigmoidocele [31]. As ultrasonography moves away from the cone, four layer structures appear, and the internal sphincter appears to be hypoechoic band, and the external sphincter muscle appears to be mixed echogenicity. Scanning the anal canal by upper, middle, and lower parts determines the structure and status of the puborectalis and the internal and external anal sphincter (Figs. 2.5 and 2.6) [32]. The importance of anal ultrasonography has been mentioned in not only the condition of cirrhosis and abscess but also in the fecal incontinence and outlet obstructive constipation. And there is a report that it can replace defecography as it can evaluate the function or internal hypertrophy from some outlet obstructive constipation patients and estimate the condition of the internal and external anal sphincter from fecal incontinence patients [31, 33]. However, as ultrasound has a significant difference to the ability of a doctor, in order to achieve an accurate result, it is important to be highly experienced.

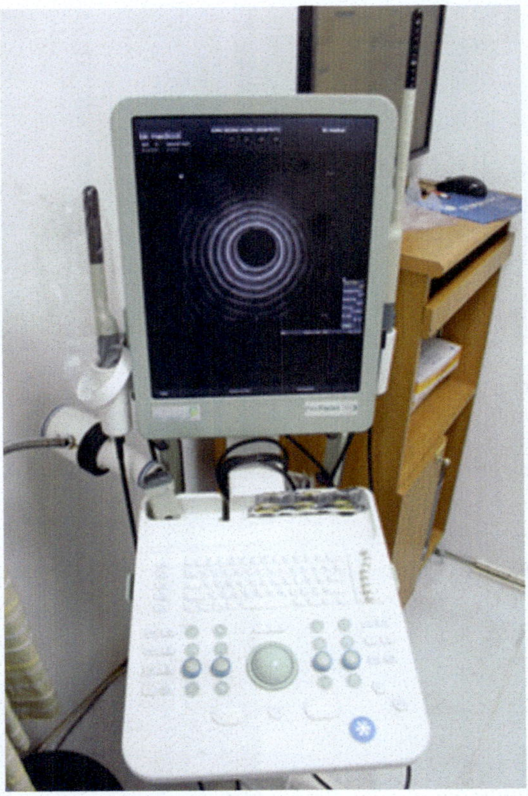

Fig. 2.4 Anorectal ultrasonography. Anal ultrasonography is the most accurate and complete testing tool for assessing structural abnormalities of an anal sphincter

The five-layered EUS model of the rectal wall, shows the alternation of hyperechoic and hypoechoic bands, the first white circle being the interface between the balloon or cap and the rectal mucosa. The second layer, black and hypoechoic, is the mucosa and superficial aspect of the submucosa. Then, the third layer, white and hyperechoic, is the interface between the submucosa and muscularis propria; a further black hypoechoic layer is the muscle layer; last, a white hyperechoic external band represents the interface with the perirectal fat.

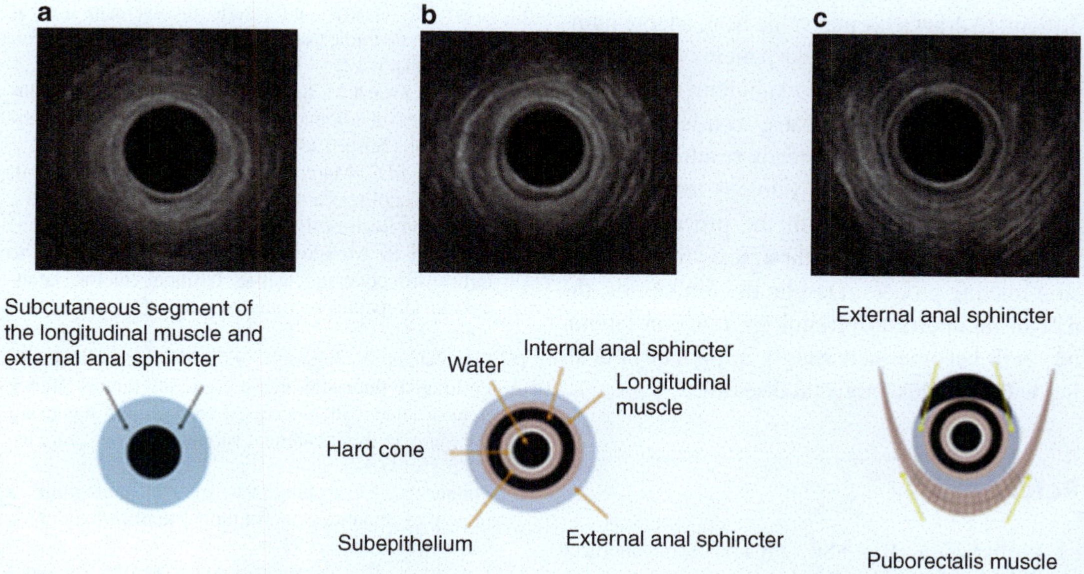

Fig. 2.5 Anal ultrasonography. The anal canal is usually divided into three levels for examination. In the lower anal canal (**a**), the echogenic external anal sphincter is seen together with the termination of the internal anal sphincter. In the middle anal canal (**b**), the internal anal sphincter is most clearly seen as a thickened hypoechoic layer. In the upper anal canal (**c**), the puborectalis muscle is seen as a U-shaped echogenic band

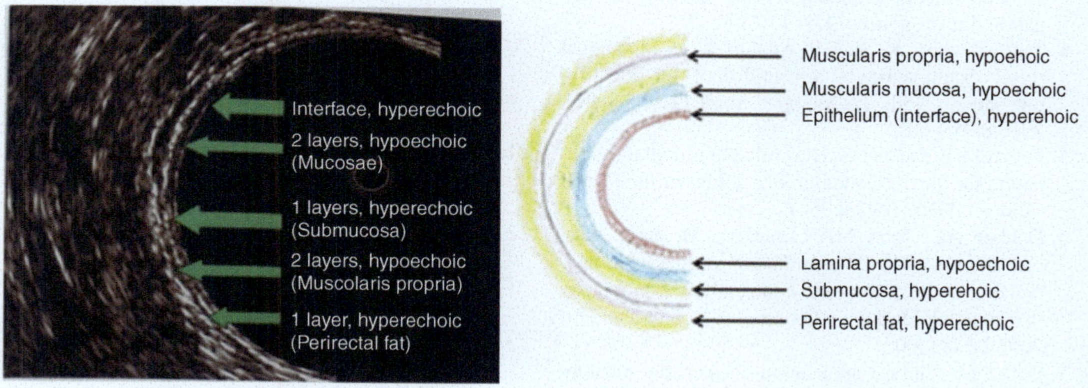

Fig. 2.6 Rectal ultrasonography

2.7 Summary

Tests performed in an anorectal physiology laboratory provide useful information for the treatment of constipation and fecal incontinence patients. Tests that are not described here can be usefully used in general experimental models. Examination area can be extended to understand the dentition, fistula, inflammatory growth disease, and postoperative functional status. The physiology laboratory can also help understand the complex correlation between the smooth muscle, rhabdomyolysis, intestinal nervous system, and hormones. In order for an anorectal physiology test to be clinically useful, the methods and the records should be standardized. However, it is difficult to draw a normal value from a large number of normal subjects, and patients with pelvic floor abnormalities tend to supplement by using other muscles or other means, so it is difficult to repeat the tests to obtain steady result. Even with easy access to anorectal physiology test, if the clinician is not familiar with the procedure, they would be hesitant to use these tests for the decision-making process. Despite the limitations, the role of an anorectal physiology function laboratory will become increasingly important in dealing with complex anorectal diseases.

References

1. Bharucha AE, Rao SSC. An update on anorectal disorders for gastroenterologists. Gastroenterology. 2014;146:37–45.
2. Bharucha AE. Recent advances in functional anorectal disorders. Curr Gastroenterol Rep. 2011;13:316–22.
3. Lam TJ, Felt-Bersma RJ. Clinical examination remains more important than anorectal function tests to identify treatable conditions in women with constipation. Int Urogynecol J. 2013;24:67–72.
4. Tantiphlachiva K, Rao P, Attaluri A, et al. Digital rectal examination is a useful tool for identifying patients with dyssynergia. Am J Gastroenterol. 2010;8:955–60.
5. Eckardt VF, Kanzler G. How reliable is digital examination for the evaluation of anal sphincter tone? Int J Colorectal Dis. 1993;8:95–7.
6. Dobben AC, Terra MP, Deutekom M, et al. Anal inspection and digital examination compared to anorectal physiology tests and endoanal ultrasonography in evaluating fecal incontinence. Int J Colorectal Dis. 2007;22:783–90.
7. Coller JA. Clinical application of anorectal manometry. Gastroenterol Clin North Am. 1987;16:17–33.
8. McHugh SM, Diamant NE. Anal canal pressure profile: a reappraisal as determined by rapid pull through technique. Gut. 1987;28:1234–41.
9. Nivatvongs S, Stern HS, Fryd DS. The length of the anal canal. Dis Colon Rectum. 1981;24:600–1.
10. Lowry AC, Simmang CL, Boulos P, Farmer KC, Finan PJ, Hyman N, et al. Consensus statement of definitions of anorectal physiology and rectal cancer. ANZ J Surg. 2001;71(10):603–5.
11. Diamant NE, Kamm MA, Wald A, Whitehead WE. AGA technical review on anorectal testing techniques. Gastroenterology. 1999;116(3):735–60.
12. Ebert EC. Gastric and enteric involvement in progressive systemic sclerosis. J Clin Gastroenterol. 2008;42(1):5–12.
13. Kiff ES, Swash M. Slowed conduction in the pudendal nerves in idiopathic (neurogenic) fecal incontinence. Br J Surg. 1984;71(8):614–6.
14. Wexner SD, Marchetti F, Salanga VD, et al. Neurophysiologic assessment of the anal sphincters. Dis Colon Rectum. 1991;34:606–12.
15. Ricciardi R, Mellgren AF, Madoff RD, et al. The utility of pudendal nerve terminal motor latencies in idiopathic incontinence. Dis Colon Rectum. 2006;49:852–7.
16. Loganathan A, Schloithe AC, Hakendorf P, et al. Prolonged pudendal nerve terminal motor latency is associated with decreased resting and squeezing pressures in the intact anal sphincter. Colorectal Dis. 2013;15:1410–5.
17. Podnar S. Electrodiagnosis of the anorectum: a review of techniques and clinical applications. Tech Coloproctol. 2003;7:71–6.
18. Lefaucher JP. Neurophysiologic testing in anorectal disorders. Muscle Nerve. 2006;33: 324–33.
19. Pfeifer J, Teoh TA, Salanga VD, Agachan F, Wexner SD. Comparative study between intra-anal sponge and needle electrode for electromyographic evaluation of constipated patients. Dis Colon Rectum. 1998;41:1153–7.
20. Axelson HW, Edebol Eeg-Olofsson K. Simplified evaluation of the paradoxical puborectalis contraction with surface electrodes. Dis Colon Rectum. 2010;53:928–31.
21. Lee BE, Kim GH. How perform and interpret balloon expulsion test. J Neurogastroenterol Motil. 2014;20:407–9.
22. Minguez M, Herreros B, Sanchiz V, et al. Predictive value of the balloon expulsion test for excluding the diagnosis of pelvic floor dyssynergia in constipation. Gastroenterology. 2004;126:57–62.
23. Bharucha AE. Update of tests of colon and rectal structure and function. J Clin Gastroenterol. 2006;40(2):96–103.
24. Rao SS, Mudipalli RS, Stressman M, et al. Investigation of the utility of colorectal function tests and Rome II criteria in dyssynergic defecation (Anismus). Neurogastroenterol Motil. 2004;16:589–96.
25. Felt-Bersma RJ, Luth WJ, Janssen II, Meuwissen SG. Defecography in patients with anorectal disorders. Dis Colon Rectum. 1990;33: 277–84.
26. Selvaggi F, Pesce G, Scotti Di Carlo E. Evaluation of normal subjects by defecographic technique. Dis Colon Rectum. 1990;33:698–702.

27. Karulf RE, Coller JA, Batolo DC, et al. Anorectal physiology testing. A survey of availability and use. Dis Colon Rectum. 1991;34:464–8.
28. Hinton JM, Lennard-Jones JE, Young AC. A mew method for studying gut transit times using radi-opaque markers. Gut. 1969;10:842–7.
29. Arhan P, Devroede G, Jehannin B, et al. Segmental colon transit time. Dis Colon Rectum. 1981;24: 625–9.
30. Metcalf AM, Phillips SF, Zinsmeister AR, MacCarty RL, Beart RW, Wolff BG. Simplified assessment of segmental colon transit. Gastroenterology. 1987;92:40–7.
31. Stoker J, Halligan S, Bartram CI. Pelvic floor imaging. Radiology. 2001;218:621–41.
32. Tjandra JJ, Milsom JW, Stolfi VM, et al. Endoluminal ultrasound defines anatomy of the anal canal and pelvic floor. Dis Colon Rectum. 1992;35:465–70.
33. Vitton V, Vignally P, Barthet M, et al. Dynamic anal endosonograpy and MRI defecography in diagnosis of pelvic floor disorders: comparison with conventional defecography. Dis Colon Rectum. 2011;54:1398–404.

Outpatient Examinations of the Anorectal Diseases

3

Jung Ryul Oh

3.1 Introduction

To examine anorectal diseases, a surgeon needs to have an enough understanding of the anatomy and a knowledge of the disease. Without patient's cooperation, an examination of the anal canal surrounded by sphincters cannot be performed. Examiner has to pay close attention to prevent unnecessary pain and fear, embarrassment, and anxiety during examination. An isolated area where patients can feel comfortable is helpful. Lithotomy position is better for relaxation of the sphincter, but in most cases, decubitus position is performed which prevents feeling shame (Fig. 3.1).

3.2 Examination Order

An examination is performed orderly by history taking, inspection, palpation, anoscopy, and proctoscopy. Palpation and anoscopy including digital rectal examination are the vital examinations.

J. R. Oh (✉)
Colorectal Division, Department of Surgery, Hansol Hospital, Seoul, South Korea

3.2.1 History Taking

As like all diseases, it is important to predict the lesion and gather enough information of symptom such as bleeding, pain, prolapse, secretion, and pruritus through detailed history taking. If a digital rectal examination is performed to the patient suspected to have anal fissure accompanied by severe pain, the patient would never want to have treatment again due to the terrible pain.

3.2.2 Inspection

Examine the perianal lesion. Check for eczema, skin tags that show the presence of anal fissure, thrombosed external hemorrhoid, incarcerated hemorrhoids, skin eruption or swelling due to abscess, and the external opening of the anal fistula (Fig. 3.2).

The lateral decubitus, or Sims position, provides optimal examination when the patient is too ill or otherwise unable to assume other positions. The patient lies on the left side with the buttocks near the edge of the examining table or bedside with the right knee and hip in slight flexion.

3.2.3 Digital Rectal Examination

Check for hardness or tenderness on pressure in the perianal by palpation. In digital rectal

D. K. Lee (ed.), *Practices of Anorectal Surgery*, https://doi.org/10.1007/978-981-13-1447-6_3

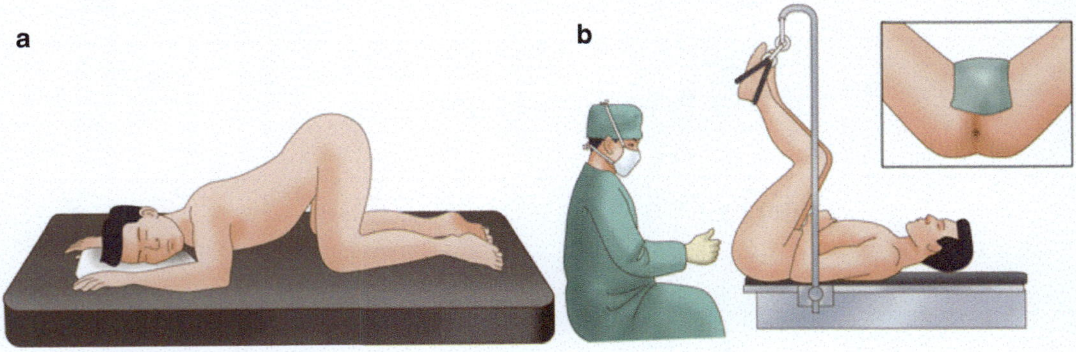

Fig. 3.1 Outpatient examination of the anorectal disease. (**a**) Knee-chest position. The proctologic (knee-chest or prone jackknife) position is the preferred position in which to examine the perineum and rectum properly. In this position, the patient can easily undergo further studies such as anoscopy and sigmoidoscopy because of easier access to the anorectum. (**b**) Lithotomy position. In the lithotomy position, the patient is supine with the legs drawn in toward the trunk and the knees allowed to fall out to the side. This position is customarily used when examining the pelvic organs in women and may offer a better examination of the anterior rectum

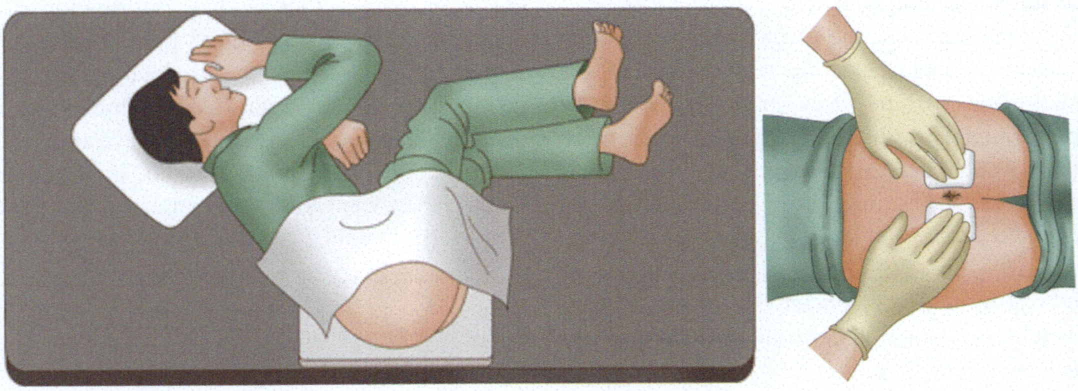

Fig. 3.2 Lateral decubitus position

examination, never insert your finger without first informing your patient with touching the perianal and making them feel comfortable in following the doctor's instruction. Put enough jelly both on the rubber gloved finger and the entrance of the anus to make it smooth for the finger to be inserted into the anal canal to check for tumor or determine the degree of hemorrhoids and ulcer. And examine by asking the patient for tenderness on pressure. Examiner can have the patient open their mouth to prevent hypertonia when inserting a finger or having the patient strain like defecation to soften the sphincter by eversion of the anal canal. If the index finger inserts smoothly, the size of the anal canal is normal. If it is difficult to insert, then the little finger is inserted to examine the degree of stenosis. An anal canal is tightened when the finger is inserted, but after 3–4 cm in length, it reaches the point where there is no resistance, and this is called the rectal ampulla. The transition from the narrow to widened part is the level of the puborectalis muscle felt at the posterior side of the anus and can be checked for relaxation by having the patient to strain like defecation. The coccyx is also felt above this area, and from the lateral, as there's pain in the sciatic nerve, the ischial spine with tenderness on pressure is also palpated. For men the prostate 6–8 cm to the center above from the anal verge is palpated, and for women, a relatively solid and movable cervix is also touched after checking for rectocele.

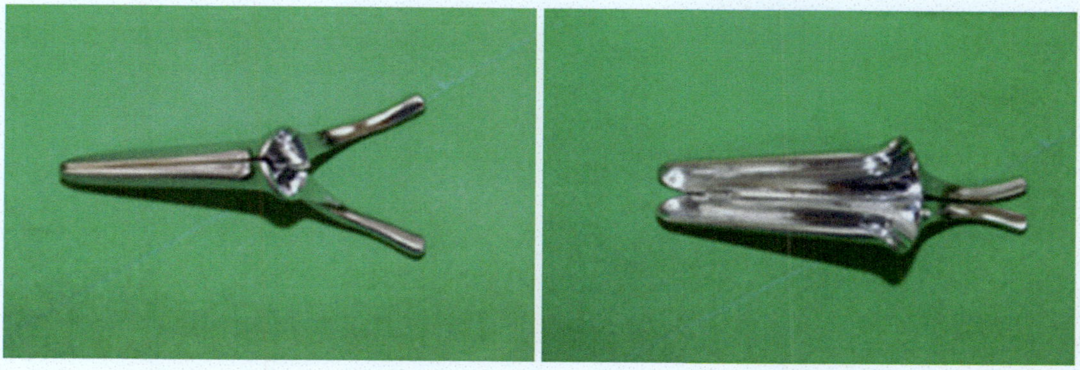

Fig. 3.3 Anoscopy

Douglas' pouch is situated on the inner side of the cervix and sometimes the bowel with stool or the ovary, and Krukenberg tumor can be checked.

3.2.4 Anoscopy

Anoscopy is divided into the one that spreads or not. Generally, the spreading one is used in outpatient clinic, which is more convenient and less painful (Fig. 3.3). Prior to using anoscopy, put lidocaine jelly on the entrance of the anus, and slightly touch the anus with anoscopy so that the patient can get used to the metallic object. After then, insert anoscopy longitudinally. With anoscopy inside, pull the skin outside the perianal of the examining area and slowly widen anoscopy. After the examination, retract the widened anoscopy, and while doing this, be cautious not to cause pain from having hair or skin caught. Repeat the process and examine the anal canal by 1/4 of the anal circumference. Proctoscopy is also used after an enema, and the patient is examined with colonoscopy for sufficient examination. Also, if necessary, biopsy can be performed.

An anoscopy is an examination using a small, rigid, tubular instrument called an anoscope (also called an anal speculum). This is inserted a few inches into the anus in order to evaluate problems of the anal canal. Anoscopy is used to diagnose hemorrhoids, anal fissures (tears in the lining of the anus), and some cancers.

3.3 Summary

When examining the anorectum, the examiner should be cautious not to have your patient feel unnecessary embarrassment, fear, anxiety, and pain, or you will not be able to achieve sufficient result. For hemorrhoid or anal fissure examination, it is done by anoscopy, and for anal fistula, it is done by digital rectal examination. Physical examination should be performed after detailed history taking to predict the disease.

Anesthesia for the Anorectal Surgery

4

Jung Ryul Oh

4.1 Introduction

Most of anal surgeries are performed under regional anesthesia, and small thrombotic hemorrhages, incision and drainage of anal abscess, and condyloma surgery can be performed under local anesthesia. There is no single anesthetic medication or anesthetic method that best suit patients. The most effective and convenient anesthetic method and medication should be used considering the patient's physical condition and age and time and site of operation. In order for a safe anesthesia, it is necessary to have sufficient knowledge and experience of anesthetic medication and method that will be used. During anesthesia and surgery, patients should be monitored continuously for changes in their vital signs using electrocardiograms, blood pressure monitors, pulse oximetry, as well as direct examination (inspection, auscultation, palpation). In preparation for emergency cases, face mask and bag for immediate use for oxygen, equipment for tracheal intubation, and emergency medicines (inotropic such as ephedrine and phenylephrine and anticholinergic drugs such as atropine) are also required.

J. R. Oh (✉)
Colorectal Division, Department of Surgery, Hansol Hospital, Seoul, South Korea

4.2 Anesthetic Method

4.2.1 Local Anesthesia

During local anesthesia, the finger is inserted into the anal canal, and subcutaneous injection is first performed, and then a needle is injected along the submucosal layer and slowly injected while identifying the injection of agent with the finger. Inject 20–40 ml each in the anterior and posterior and on both sides of the anus. In local anesthesia, lidocaine, mepivacaine, and bupivacaine are usually used. Lidocaine shows effect within 2–5 minutes after injection. It has fast action time but short duration of 1–2 hours, but if mixture of epinephrine is used 1:200,000, it can last up to 4 hours. The maximum dose of lidocaine is 200 mg, and when mixed with vasoconstrictor, it is 500 mg. The maximum dose of mepivacaine is 500 mg. Bupivacaine is chemically similar to mepivacaine, but its anesthetic action is four times stronger than mepivacaine or lidocaine, and its duration is two to three times longer. It is used for longer anesthesia, for 0.25% submucosal anesthesia about 200 minutes, and for 0.25–0.5% neural block or epidural block about 3–6 hours. The maximum dosage is 175 mg, and if mixed with vasoconstrictor, it is 225 mg. As with other local anesthetics, side effects such as convulsions, circulatory collapse, and myocardial inhibitory activity can be occurred.

D. K. Lee (ed.), *Practices of Anorectal Surgery*, https://doi.org/10.1007/978-981-13-1447-6_4

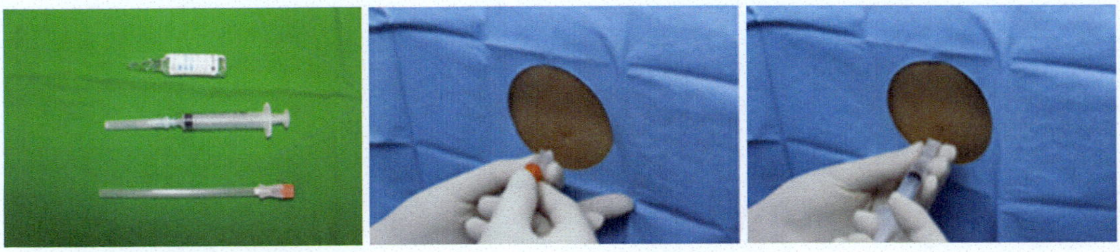

Fig. 4.1 Spinal anesthesia

4.2.2 Regional Anesthesia

Regional anesthesia performed in anal surgery is spinal and caudal anesthesia. It is widely used because it can relax the pelvic muscles enough to perform a wide range of anal surgery such as incarcerated hemorrhoids or horseshoe abscess without difficulty. Spinal anesthesia is a method of injecting local anesthetic into the subarachnoid space which may result in headache due to dural damage and voiding difficulty (Fig. 4.1). Rare but complications from spinal nerve injury can occur. Caudal anesthesia is a type of epidural anesthesia, and there is no risk of perforation of the dura resulting in complication of headache after anesthesia. However, systemic toxicity can lead to severe complications such as dyspnea and loss of consciousness. And it is not recommended to use this method if you are not experienced as drugs should be injected into a narrow space. In caudal anesthesia, about 10–30 mg of lidocaine, 3.5–7 mg of bupivacaine, 5–10 mg of ropivacaine, and as anesthesia adjuvant 10–25 ug of fentanyl do not delay the sensory and motor nerve recovery [1].

4.2.3 Monitored Anesthesia Care

A monitored anesthesia care is the so-called hypno-anesthesia, in which a sedative-analgesic drug is used as intravenous injection. Monitoring anesthesia care can be used in combination with local anesthesia or regional anesthesia to improve patient satisfaction and shorten recovery time rather than being used independently [2]. The most common approach is to use sedatives, midazolam (1–3 mg) and propofol (25–100 ug/kg/min), in combination with narcotic analgesics [3]. Recently, the use of dexmedetomidine (0.5–1 ug/kg) and ketamine (75–150 ug/kg) has been increasing as they can reduce the incidence of respiratory depression caused by the use of sedative-analgesic [4]. Respiratory depression is caused by excessive sedation; therefore, it requires special attention for the medical team when conducting the surgery.

4.3 Complications

4.3.1 Complications Followed by the Use of Local Anesthetic

Patients who respond sensitively to pain may have vasovagal attack after injection. After anal local anesthetic, temporary loss of consciousness, nausea, vomiting, pale, bradycardia, or hypotension may occur in 1 out of 1000 patients. For the treatment, position patient in Trendelenburg's position and administer oxygen. If bradycardia persists, 1 mg of atropine may be injected.

When high concentration of local anesthetic is used, due to central nervous system toxicity, drowsiness, tinnitus, abnormal sense of the tongue and mouth area, visual disturbance, muscle tremor, unconsciousness, and paralysis may occur. Also due to cardiovascular toxicity, circulatory collapse and cardiac arrest may occur. For the treatment, administer oxygen, and in the case of seizure, 10 mg of diazepam is administered.

4.3.2 Headache Due to Dural Damage

In spinal anesthesia, if intracranial pressure changes with having spinal fluid flows through the area where the injection needle is punctured, then the pain-sensitive dural sac structure will shift which causes headache. It can be diagnosed by its typical symptoms. Symptoms are improved when lying down, but it gets worse when standing or moving, and it appears to have high frequency in younger patients. The thicker the needle, the higher the probability of occurrence. In the past, when a thick 19G needle was used, the incidence was as high as 70%, but recently it has been reported that thin 23G needles are used, and the incidence is around 3–16%. As for the needle shape, there is a report that pencil-shaped needles reduce the incidence. And as for cutting the needle, frequent puncturing can increase dural puncture damage [5]. To reduce the incidence, needle angle is important. The incidence is high when the needle is used in vertical angle [6]. There's also a report that after the puncture, by reinserting the stylet when the needle is retreated, it can reduce the incidence of headache to 5% from 16% [7].

There is no definite evidence in reducing the pain from dural puncture by a good bed rest and fluid supply, and the efficacy of anesthesia by the patient's position is also uncertain.

Treatments are mainly conservative treatment, such as bed rest, fluid supply, and analgesic treatment. Headache usually improves within 72 hours to 7 days after conservative treatment. However, there is no definite evidence in reducing the pain from dural puncture by bed rest and fluid supply. Hydrocortisone is considered to reduce intensity of headache by sodium and fluid retention, and it has been reported that intravenous administration of dexamethasone resulted in less headaches after spinal anesthesia (2.5% vs 12.5%) [8]. However, with severe symptoms, conservative treatment won't work, and autologous blood patch works the most effective, which sealed off the punctured site of the dural fiber with autologous blood. It is reported that 20–30 ml of autologous blood is collected and immediately injected slowly into the epidural space and the symptoms improved to 70–98% [9].

4.4 Summary

When determining the operation, it is important to evaluate the overall patient condition, including the patient's medical history and family history, and also the selection of the operation method. The choice of anesthetic considering the patient condition and type of operation effects is an important factor to the patient's recovery and discharge from hospital. By choosing appropriate anesthetic method, it will minimize postoperative complications and return the patients to their daily life with early discharge.

References

1. Ben-David B, Maryanovsky M, Gurevitch A, Lucyk C, Solosko D, Frankel R, et al. A comparison of minidose lidocaine-fentanyl and conventional-dose lidocaine spinal anesthesia. Anesth Analg. 2000;91(4):865–70.
2. Sa Rego MM, Watcha MF, White PF. The changing role of monitored anesthesia care in the ambulatory setting. Anesth Analg. 1997;85(5):1020–36.
3. Taylor E, Ghouri AF, White PF. Midazolam in combination with propofol for sedation during local anesthesia. J Clin Anesth. 1992;4(3):213–6.
4. Arain SR, Ebert TJ. The efficacy, side effects, and recovery characteristics of dexmedetomidine versus propofol when used for intraoperative sedation. Anesth Analg. 2002;95(2):461–6, table of contents.
5. Xu H, Liu Y, Song W, Kan S, Liu F, Zhang D, et al. Comparison of cutting and pencil-point spinal needle in spinal anesthesia regarding postdural puncture headache: a meta-analysis. Medicine (Baltimore). 2017;96(14):e6527.
6. Richman JM, Joe EM, Cohen SR, Rowlingson AJ, Michaels RK, Jeffries MA, et al. Bevel direction and postdural puncture headache: a meta-analysis. Neurologist. 2006;12(4):224–8.
7. Strupp M, Brandt T, Muller A. Incidence of post-lumbar puncture syndrome reduced by reinserting the stylet: a randomized prospective study of 600 patients. J Neurol. 1998;245(9):589–92.
8. Hamzei A, Basiri-Moghadam M, Pasban-Noghabi S. Effect of dexamethasone on incidence of headache after spinal anesthesia in cesarean section. A single blind randomized controlled trial. Saudi Med J. 2012;33(9):948–53.
9. Turnbull DK, Shepherd DB. Post-dural puncture headache: pathogenesis, prevention and treatment. Br J Anaesth. 2003;91(5):718–29.

5 Hemorrhoids

Gyu Young Jeong

5.1 Introduction

The pathophysiology of the hemorrhoids had been ambiguous for long until the definition was clearly defined as vascular cushions in 1975 by Thomson [1]. Thick spongy submucosa in anal canal is not usually hemorrhoid but anal cushion formed at submucosa by overlapping of superior hemorrhoidal artery and middle hemorrhoidal artery (hemorrhoidal plexus). There are not only vessels but also muscular fibers in anal cushion. Muscular fibers are based in conjoined longitudinal muscle and internal sphincter, and attach the cushion to the internal sphincter (Fig. 5.1). The cushion is dilated with blood when defecating and protects the internal sphincter. Internal hemorrhoidal plexus is contributed by superior hemorrhoidal artery and middle hemorrhoidal artery. And external hemorrhoidal plexus is supplied by inferior hemorrhoidal artery. The vein is drained to superior, middle, and inferior hemorrhoidal vein.

5.2 Pathophysiology

There are several hypotheses on the occurrence of hemorrhoids. Some are circulation disorder caused by hypertrophy and congestion of the anal cushion, sliding down of the anal cushion, tearing of the supporting tissue of the anal cushion, and abnormal dilatation of the vessel of the internal hemorrhoidal plexus. Others that are related to the occurrence of hemorrhoids are genetic, age, anal sphincter pressure, dietary habits, job, constipation, pregnancy, etc. [2]. The most reliable hypothesis is considered to be the sliding theory that the hemorrhoids occur due to having supporting muscular fiber tissue of hemorrhoidal plexus get worse or loss of elasticity from the tearing (Fig. 5.2).

5.3 Classification

Hemorrhoids above the dentate line are internal hemorrhoids, and they are usually covered with rectal mucosa. Hemorrhoids below the dentate line are external hemorrhoids, and they are wrapped around with squamous epithelium. Coexisted internal and external hemorrhoids that occured passing through up and down the dentate line are called mixed hemorrhoids. Internal hemorrhoids can be classified into 1 to 4 grades by the degree of prolapse (Fig. 5.3).

5.4 Diagnosis

When examining the patient for diagnosis, it has to be done comfortably with giving detail explanation on the process, so that the patient does not

G. Y. Jeong (✉)
Colorectal Division, Department of Surgery, Hansol Hospital, Seoul, South Korea

D. K. Lee (ed.), *Practices of Anorectal Surgery*, https://doi.org/10.1007/978-981-13-1447-6_5

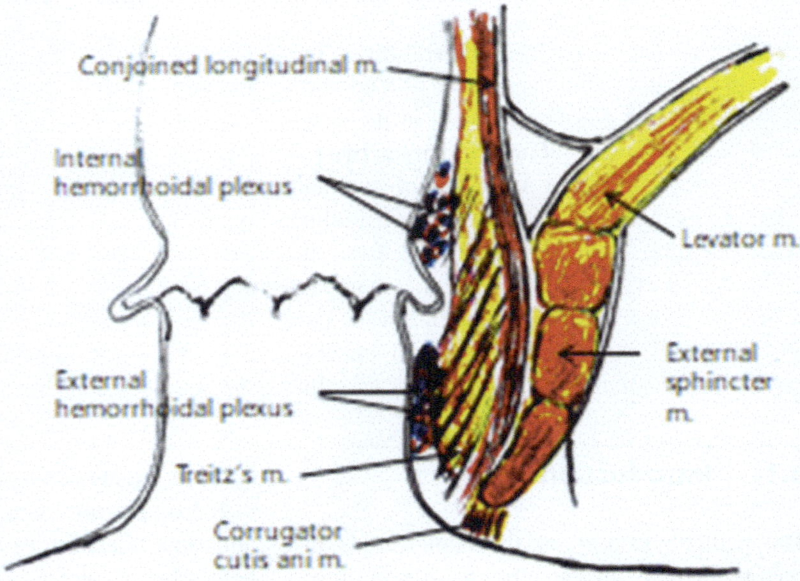

Fig. 5.1 Relationship of the hemorrhoidal plexus with conjoined longitudinal muscle. Muscular fibers are based in conjoined longitudinal muscle and internal sphincter, and attach the cushion to internal sphincter. The cushion is dilated with blood when defecating, and protects internal sphincter

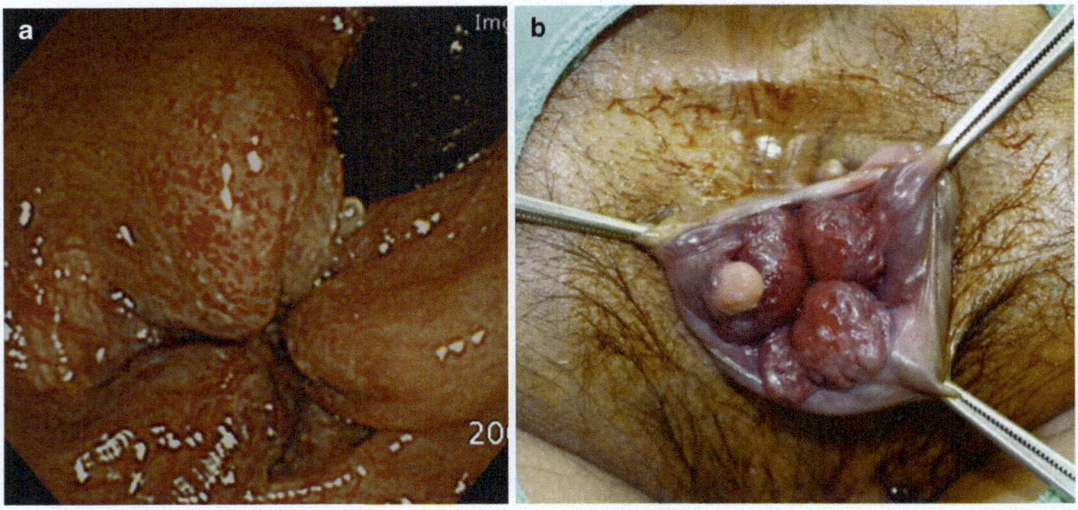

Fig. 5.2 Findings of hemorrhoids. (**a**) Colonoscopic view of the anorectal area after retroversion of the scope in the rectum. Internal hemorrhoids are noted. (**b**) External view of the anus in the same patient. Internal hemorrhoids are protruding

feel disconcerted. The most important thing in diagnosing hemorrhoids is the history taking. The most common symptoms of patients with hemorrhoids are bleeding and prolapse. They have clear bright red blood drops or, in severe cases, blood pistol. The bleeding occurs generally in the internal hemorrhoids and can be accompanied by anemia. Degree of prolapse can guide you to choosing the treatment, and if the prolapse continues, there could be pruritus ani. Hemorrhoids without complications do not have pain, but thrombus, ulcer, and incarcerated hemorrhoids have severe pain and discomfort. It can be diagnosed by careful inspection, palpation, and digital examination for necessary physical examination [3, 4]. Anorectal physiology tests do not help to diagnose hemorrhoids; however, it can help predict the possibility of postoperative

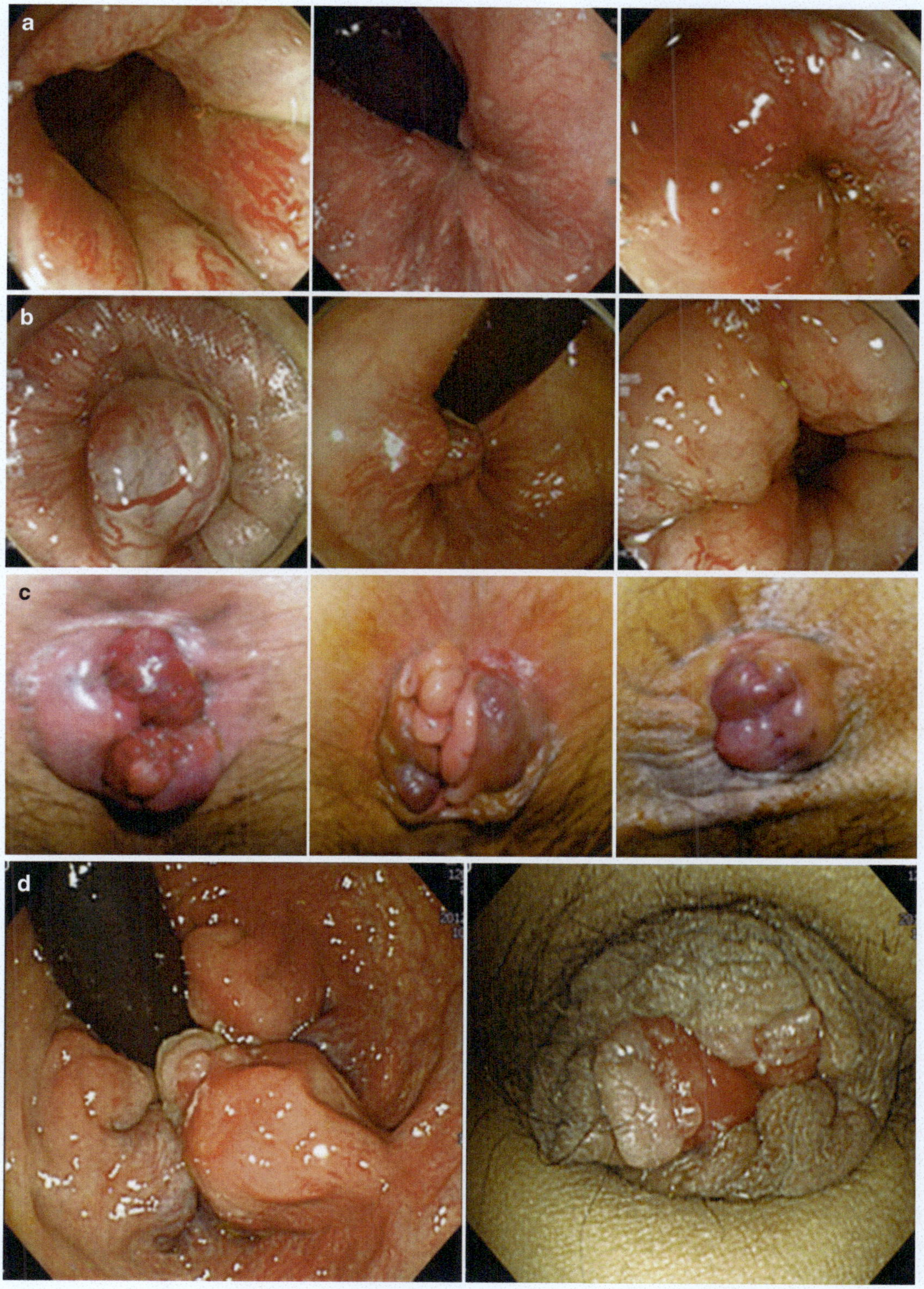

Fig. 5.3 Classification of internal hemorrhoids. (**a**) First-degree hemorrhoids (gradeI): The anal cushions bleed but do not prolapse. (**b**) Second-degree hemorrhoids (grade II): The anal cushions prolapse through the anus on straining but reduce spontaneously. (**c**) Third-degree hemorrhoids (grade III): The anal cushions prolapse through the anus on straining or exertion and require manual replacement into the anal canal. (**d**) Fourth-degree hemorrhoids (grade IV): The prolapse stays out at all times and is irreducible

fecal incontinence and check for accompanied sphincter function. Also, through sufficient inspection, palpation, and digital examination, it helps a lot in distinguishing whether it is accompanying Crohn's disease, anal fissure or thrombosed hemorrhoids, abscess, or tumorous lesion. Hemorrhoids may be suspected by the color of blood and the appearance of bleeding; however, colonoscopic examination is vital for those who are in the age of colon cancer screening or have family history of cancer [5].

5.5 Treatment

A number of hemorrhoids treatments have been introduced and used and also many of them disappeared. In order to choose an appropriate treatment, it is most important to have clear understanding of hemorrhoid pathophysiology. Traditionally, treatment of hemorrhoids is based on the degree of prolapse, severity of symptom, and appearance of the hemorrhoids. In general cases, it can be treated as outpatient; however, it can differ from considering the patient's preference and international insurance conditions and also from the experience of the doctor. It is not easy to set standard guideline for the outpatient treatment diseases including hemorrhoids.

5.5.1 Dietary and Life style Modification

The key factors of conservative treatment are the dietary habits and lifestyle change. Constipation is the main factor for hemorrhoids, as it makes the patient sit in the toilet for long time and strain strongly for defecation. Therefore, it is important to treat constipation. Have patient drink sufficient amount of water and obtain food that has a lot of fiber or commercialized fiber [6, 7]. It is advisable to have them take probiotics, as one of the reasons people hesitate in obtaining fiber is gas and sense of abdominal discomfort. In rare cases, stool can become solid after taking fiber, therefore hyperosmolar laxatives like lactulose may need to be administered together. The treatment should continue at least 6 weeks to be effective. Warm sitz bath can improve blood circulation which can reduce the size of dilated hemorrhoidal plexus and can stop the bleeding at defecation by having hypertonic sphincter relax. Put anus in warm water 2–3 times a day each time about 5–10 minutes. Sometimes, cold pack is recommended for thrombosed hemorrhoids, but warm sitz bath is more effective. It is important that the patients do not drink alcohol during the treatment, as alcohol dilates vessel and, in some cases, relates to diarrhea which worsens symptom of hemorrhoids.

5.5.2 Medical Treatment

In order to improve symptoms of hemorrhoids, there are many commercial topical agents such as cream, lotion, suppository, and local anesthesia, and it is hard to prove the effectiveness, but it is often used out of experience. Local medication is classified into ointment, suppository, and oral medication. Local medication acts in elevating lymph drainage, increasing permeability of capillary, and strengthening blood vessel wall, efficacy of local anesthesia, and anti-inflammatory action. It is more effective in treating 1 or 2 degrees of hemorrhoids that has bleeding, and in the case of prolapse, it is not so effective [8]. Suppository or ointment is not easy to put or insert in the exact area. Many patients insert suppository too deep or put ointment in perianal area. With the medical treatment, dietary and lifestyle modification should be combined to be effective.

5.5.3 Invasive procedure

In the past, manual dilatation (Lord's procedure, 1968) and cryotherapy were used; however, it is no longer in use as it has risk of fecal incontinence. The most used invasive procedure is rubber band ligation. Others are sclerotherapy and infrared coagulation, but rubber band ligation is generally known for the outstanding result [9].

5.5.3.1 Rubber Band Ligation

Rubber band ligation (1954) is commonly used for internal hemorrhoid treatment, and as it does not usually require anesthesia, many patients with need of surgical treatment have been replaced with this procedure [10, 11]. The principle is, by using specially designed ligator to tie the hemorrhoidal plexus, it will fall out with ischemic and necrosis, and ulcer will form, but, as scar appears during the healing process, it gets fixed on the rectal wall (Fig. 5.4). The technique is simple, but if it is ligated below the dentate line, the pain is severe; therefore hemorrhoidal plexus should be ligated at approximately 2cm above the dentate line. After enema, insert proctoscopy to identify hemorrhoidal plexus before ligation. It is possible to ligate two to three piles at a time; however, it is recommended to ligate one pile first and check progress of the healing and perform the next ligation after 1 month. It is said that it can be ligated three at a time, but if possible, ligating only up to two at a time is recommended [12]. After the ligation, fiber and stool softener should be administered. This treatment modality does not have many complications; however, it can have pelvic inflammation, so antibiotics should be prescribed for the first day after the procedure. Also, after the ligation, thrombus can occur in external hemorrhoid, so warm sitz bath should be recommended. And like hemorrhoidectomy, patients should be informed that 2% of the treated patients may have bleeding before and after the first week as the strangulated tissue sloughs. For those who administer anticoagulant drugs should not have this treatment, as it can cause bleeding from 25% of those who administer warfarin and 7% of those who administer other anticoagulant drugs like aspirin [13]. Recurrence rate is reported variously between 11% and 49%, but the advantage is that it can be treated again easily when recurred [9, 14]. Band ligation, with simple manipulation and low expense, and as it can be widely used without anesthesia in one to three internal piles, has high satisfaction from the patients. But realistically in Korea, it has difficulty on the management side of the hospital to use this as a single treatment due to the medical insurance system.

5.5.3.2 Sclerotherapy

It can be applied in internal hemorrhoids with 1 to 3 degrees, but generally, it is selectively performed to the patient who is not applicable to have band ligation treatment with 1- or 2-degree hemorrhoids or who has coagulation disorder. The used sclerotic agent varies by the countries, but 5% phenol in almond oil has been used the most [15]. Recently in Japan, excellent results were reported by using Zion injection (aluminum potassium sulfate in tannic acid) for sclerotherapy [16, 17]. It was once popularly used also in Korea, but it is no longer in use due to the problem with supply and insurance fee. The principle of the treatment is, by injecting sclerotic agent in

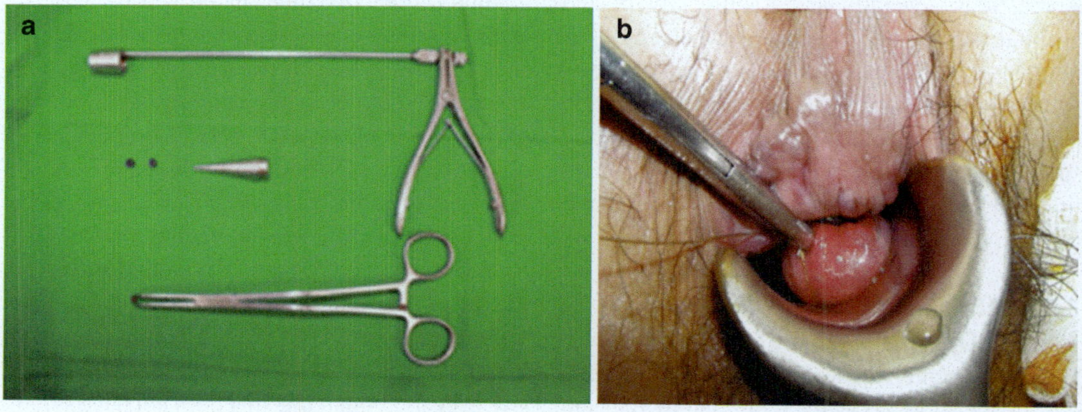

Fig. 5.4 Rubber band ligation. (**a**) McGivney type ligator. (**b**) Hemorrhoidal plexus should be ligated above the dentate line

submucosal layer, the tissue gets fixed by vasoconstriction and coagulation and fibrosis. The results have been reported variously and, like the band ligation, rare, but severe complications such as prostate abscess and retroperitoneal abscess may occur, so prophylactic antibiotic injection is necessary [18, 19].

5.5.3.3 Infrared Coagulation

The principle of the treatment is using infrared rays directly on hemorrhoids causes necrosis of protein within the hemorrhoids. This is used generally in 1- or 2-degree hemorrhoids and can be used again when recurred. Recent reports have similar results as band ligation; however, it is not generally used for 3- or 4-degree hemorrhoids. Due to the medical insurance system, it is barely used in Korea [20, 21].

5.5.4 Operative Treatment

Excisional hemorrhoidectomy is applied to the cases accompanied by external hemorrhoids, ulcer, incarceration and strangulation, widespread thrombosis, hypertrophic papilla, anal fissure, or in the case of failed treatment with rubber band ligation. It is outstanding treatment for 3- to 4-degree hemorrhoids compared to the nonoperative treatment [9]. In western countries like the USA and Europe, hemorrhoids operation could be treated under local anesthesia and light hypnoanesthesia in the outpatient department. But in Korea, it is generally and traditionally treated hospitalized and under spinal anesthesia. This is to reduce anxiety from the patients and also better for postoperative management. Operation position can be decided by the preference of the surgeon, whether prone jack knife position or lithotomy position, but we prefer prone jack knife position to avoid the discomfort of assistant.

5.5.4.1 Excisional Hemorrhoidectomy (Open and Closed)

Excisional hemorrhoidectomy has various methods, by the surgeon, by the tools, and by the generation, but the most generally used methods nowadays are excision and ligation hemorrhoidectomy and hemorrhoidopexy using auto-stapler device. Excising and ligating the stump of hemorrhoidal pile is one of the most widely used methods in the world. 1:200,000 epinephrine mixed distilled water is injected on submucosal layer of excising hemorrhoid and start excising after 2–3 minutes. Submucous injection can reduce bleeding and can separate hemorrhoidal plexus easier from the internal sphincter. Including external hemorrhoid, hold the skin which will be excised with forceps, and pull up and draw excisional line using scalpel. Then using scalpel or Metzenbaum scissors, start excision with being cautious not to have excise subcutaneous external sphincter as it is closely attached with the external hemorrhoids. Part of muscular fiber from conjoined longitudinal muscle penetrates the internal sphincter and gets attached to the hemorrhoidal plexus, and the blood vessel. The muscular fiber appears tense when hemorrhoidal plexus is pulled during the operation. By cutting the tense muscular fibers selectively, the hemorrhoidal plexus can be separated easily without damaging internal sphincter. In this procedure, the know-how is using Metzenbaum scissors with dull edge than sharp one, as it can reduce bleeding caused by injuries of blood vessel. From anal verge, excision range should not be wider than 1 cm and should be narrower as it goes through the anal canal. When the dissection is completed, absorbable suture thread is used to ligate, using 2-0 or 3-0 chromic catgut as it does not slip and it is easy to ligate. Most ligation is done two times in a row (Fig. 5.5). An excision order usually starts from the left side of anus, but in the case of big hemorrhoid, it is prioritized. When excising hemorrhoidal pile in posterior side of the anus, it is recommended to minimize the excision range. In bowel movement, the pressure is high to posterior side of the anus, which makes delayed healing of the postoperative wound; therefore, the wound should be minimized or sutured. If possible, excised pile should not exceed four piles, and it is important to prevent narrowing of the anus caused by excessive excision. Small pile that does not have symptom can be left, and treated outpatient later under local anesthesia. There can be different results to

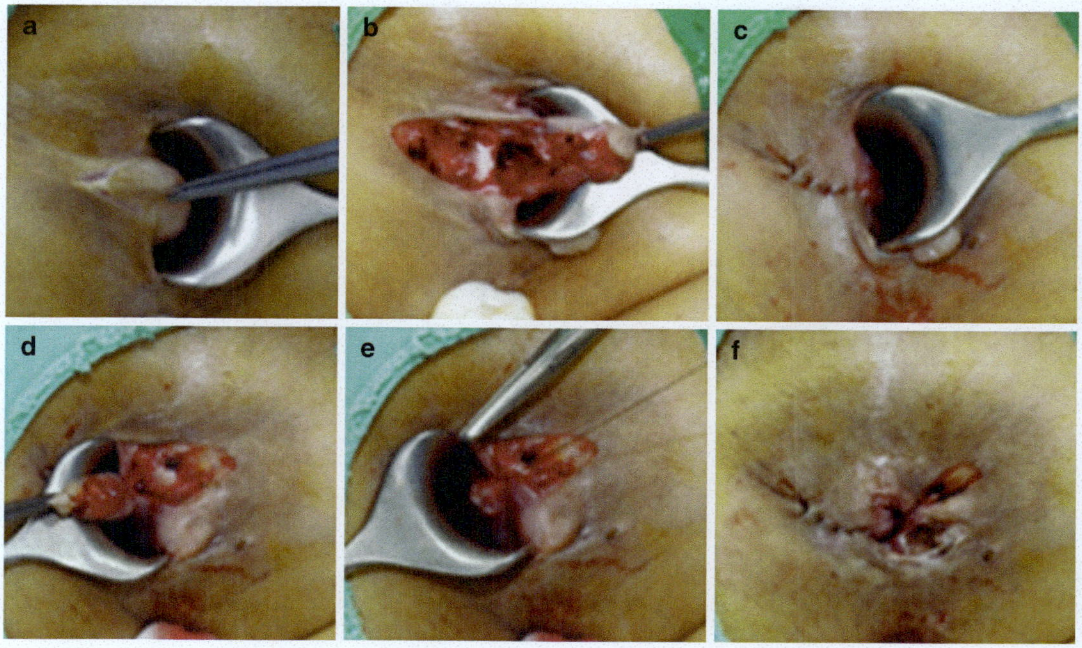

Fig. 5.5 Excisional hemorrhoidectomy. (**a**) Including external hemorrhoid, hold the skin which will be excised with forceps, and pull up and draw excisional line using scalpel. (**b**) Then using scalpel or Metzenbaum scissor, start excision with being cautious not to have the excision margin follow subcutaneous external sphincter as it is closely attached with external hemorrhoid. Including external hemorrhoid, hold the skin which will be excised with forceps, and pull up and draw excisional line using scalpel. (**c**) There can be different results to leaving the wound open. This is closed method. (**d**) In the open method, inital procedures are the same as above. (**e**) 2-0 chromic catgut is generally used to ligate the stump. (**f**) Open method and closed method are mixed

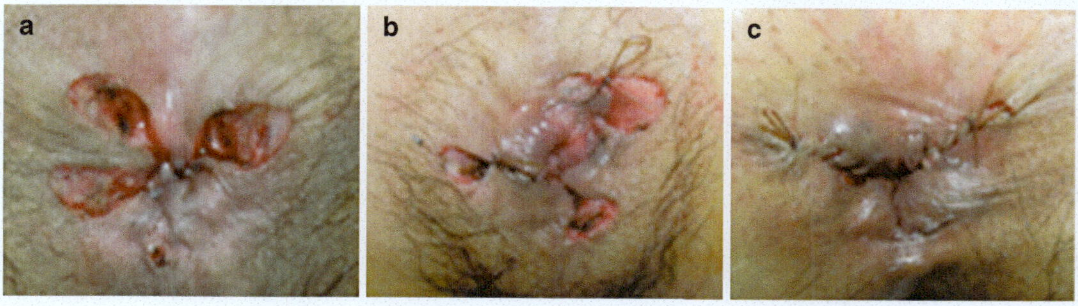

Fig. 5.6 Three different methods to manage the wound. (**a**) Open method, Milligan-Morgan hemorrhoidectomy. (**b**) Semiclosed method. (**c**) Closed method, Ferguson hemorrhoidectomy

leaving the wound closed [22] or open [23] after excision (Fig. 5.6). Whether to use closed or open method should be decided prior to the operation. Semiclosed method has been also widely used [24]. 3-0 or 4-0 chromic catgut is generally used to suture wound for the closed or semiclosed method. Generally, closed method results in faster wound healing and less pain, and it is known to have less complication [25–27], and the author had same results in the prospective randomized study.

Some surgeons prefer semiclosed method, suturing anal mucosa and leaving outer side of anal verge open. Whichever method surgeons use, the result is acceptable, so it is recommended to use preferred method. In case of incarcerated circumferential hemorrhoids with severe pain, just excise three to four hemorrhoidal plexus

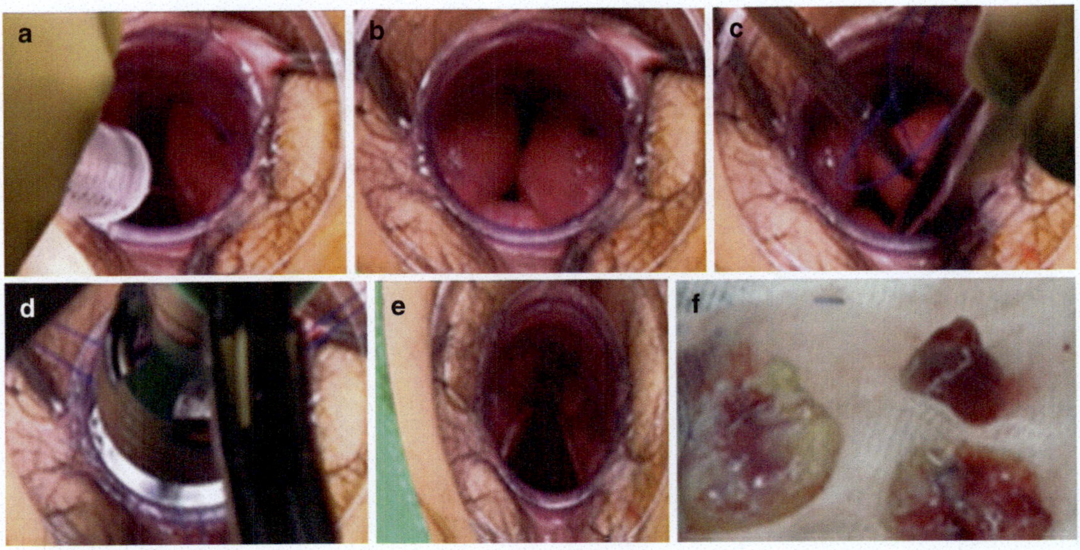

Fig. 5.7 Partial stapled hemorrhoidectomy. (**a**) Mixed epinephrine and lidocaine are injected to avoid firing pain. (**b**) Appearance of the swollen mucous membrane. (**c**) Purse-string suture with nonabsorbable suture. (**d**) Firing with stapler. (**e**) After fired, three mucosal bridges should be cut. (**f**) Resected specimens

that has the biggest thrombus and incise in between the accessory piles and remove only the thrombus or leave as it is. In patients with high anal pressure in resting period, lateral internal sphincterotomy is no more used separately, as it has no advantage compared to excisional hemorrhoidectomy with sphincterotomy. There are several reports that bipolar energy device, LigaSure, or Harmonic scalpel has less pain when used for hemorrhoid excision; however, due to high expense, it is not generally used in Korea [28–30].

5.5.4.2 Procedure for Prolapsed Hemorrhoids (PPH)

PPH was invented by Doctor Longo in 1998; based on the rationale, the cause of the hemorrhoids is from a sliding theory of anal cushion, which makes superior/middle hemorrhoid blood vessels stretch and distort. Therefore, by blocking of the blood flow of the superior hemorrhoid blood vessels and pulling up prolapsed anorectal mucosa placing anal cushion in place will shrink the hemorrhoids [31]. Generally it is used for 3- or 4-degree internal hemorrhoids and can be excised in parallel with the external hemorrhoids or skin tags if necessary. Some external hemorrhoids go into anal canal automatically after the operation, and as time passes, it shrinks and symptoms disappear. In second-degree internal hemorrhoid, rubber band ligation is more simple and convenient treatment than PPH.

PPH consists of a circular stapler, a suture threader, a circular anal dilator, and a purse-string anoscope. The surgical technique is to use nonabsorbable suture thread and purse-string suture mucosa including submucosa in the 2–4 cm above the dentate line. Be cautious not to suture the muscular layer or vagina in the case of women patients. The site of purse-string suture is well above (at least 2 cm above the dentate line) to prevent anal mucosa and anal internal sphincter getting into the suture line. If it is not prevented, severe postoperative pain may occur. In order to perform suture in a proper position, use electrocautery to make a round mark around the suturing site before inserting anoscopy. Also, if suture line is too far above, prolapsed hemorrhoid will still be remained after the operation. After firing of the stapler, wait about 1 minute before releasing; then there will be almost no anastomotic bleeding. Recently, suturing only hemorrhoidal piles selectively and excision operation is used rather than using purse-string suture on all rectal mucosa (Fig. 5.7) [32–34].

Compared to the other existing operation, PPH has less pain and shorter period of hospitalization, which makes the patient return to their daily life faster [35, 36]. While excision and ligation method have a sharp and severe pain, PPH has rather dull pain or heavy feeling. The postoperative complications are similar as existing operation, but in rare cases, severe inflammation could occur around the pelvic cavity and retroperitoneum [37], and as of today, four death cases have been reported [38]. Therefore it is safe to inject intravenous antibiotics before and after the operation. There also have been cases with rectovaginal fistula occurrence; to prevent this, be cautious not to have vaginal wall go into suturing line during purse-string suturing. Stapled hemorrhoidopexy is less pain than excisional hemorrhoidectomy, but it is reported to have over 30% of recurrence rate based on the 10-year long-term follow-up reports. There is a controversy in the cause of postoperative recurrence, however, based on the pathogenesis of the vascular hyperplasia, there is actually no block of blood flow after PPH [39, 40]. It may make the recurrence rate higher than the excision and ligation operation in third or fourth hemorrhoids. In my experience, after completion of the PPH procedure, if anastomotic line is excessively above the dentate line, pain is less but recurrence rate is higher. Therefore, it is recommended to have anastomotic line within 1 cm above the dentate line.

5.6 Postoperative Complications

5.6.1 Pain

Pain is one of the main reasons patients hesitate to take surgery of the hemorrhoids. Postoperative pain is related to the degree of hemorrhoids, patient's pain sensitivity, and surgical techniques. Excessive excision can cause long-term ripping pain during bowel movement. Sphincter damage and ligation during surgery can cause pain from sphincter spasm after defecation. The pain is severe and lasts long period; therefore, it is important to be cautious not to partially ligate the sphincter muscle during operation. There have been various studies and attempts to reduce postoperative pain, and one of them is known to reduce pain due to spasm of the sphincter muscle by partial incision in the internal sphincter, but there is high risk in having flatus incontinence [41]. However, the author also combines partial incision if determined during the operation that there could be severe postoperative pain or postoperative stenosis due to severe hemorrhoids. Injecting Botox or bupivacaine at the end of the operation is known to reduce postoperative pain [42–44]. To reduce spasm in internal sphincter after the operation, use diltiazem or GTN ointment, which is known to reduce pain [45–47]. Nowadays, most patients use PCA (patient controlled analgesia) after operation for the pain management and prescribed anti-inflammatory analgesic drug. As postoperative constipation can cause excessive straining which worsens the severity of pain, fiber and stool softener can be administered to facilitate defecation. But if diarrhea occurs due to stool softener, this may rather worsen the pain due to anal hypertonicity, so it is important not to have diarrhea. There is controversy whether antibiotics help postoperative pain control, but it is selectively used in the patients with high risk of infection or PPH operated patients [48].

5.6.2 Urinary Retention

About 10% of the patients have postoperative urinary retention, and this is one of the main disruptive factors in a day surgery and mainly occurs in the elderly men. The causing factors of urinary retention are spinal anesthesia, excessive fluid, gauze packing in the anal canal, rectal pain, and spasm [49, 50]. If there is no voiding 8 hours after the surgery, the bladder has to be emptied using catheter. It will help to have the warm water running on the anus and try voiding by pressing the abdomen downward from the umbilicus using both hands.

5.6.3 Postoperative Bleeding

There are two kinds of postoperative bleeding, one immediately after the operation and the other

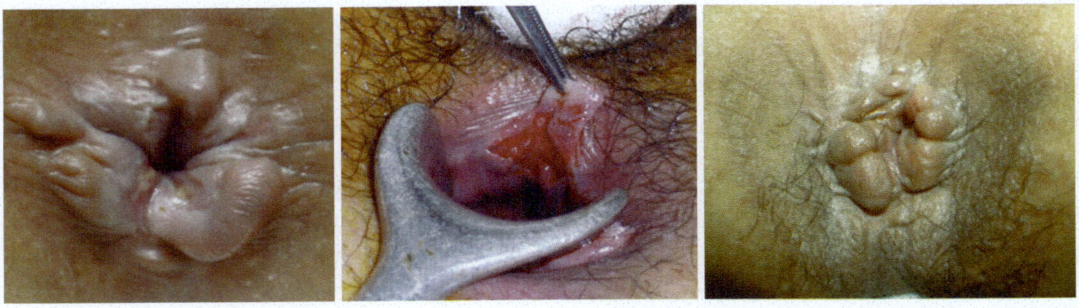

Fig. 5.8 Delayed wound healing, anal fissure, and stenosis with skin tags after hemorrhoidectomy

1–2 weeks after the operation. From the bleeding which occurs immediately after the operation, the bleeding from wound may be stopped with pressure, but the bleeding from the internal anus mostly is massive bleeding, and from ligated site of the stump, the bleeding site has to be identified and ligated in the operation room immediately. Delayed hemorrhage incidence is about 1%, and the distinctive symptom is that the patients feel bowel movement with bubbling and have massive dark red blood like diarrhea. In severe cases, patients can faint and suffer from dizziness. Prior to discharging the patient, it is necessary to inform and educate patient with delayed hemorrhage, and if this occurs, they have to come to the hospital immediately. And in this case, with the arrival to the hospital, fluid should be supplied, and bleeding site has to be ligated in the operation room. A surgeon has to be aware that hemorrhage may occur even during the use of hemostatic agent. Bleeding area cannot be identified due to decreasing blood pressure which stops bleeding naturally, but delayed hemorrhage should be identified visually as possible, and if the bleeding area is not clear, hemostatic gauze should be placed in the anal canal.

5.6.4 Delayed Wound Healing and Anal Stenosis

The most common postoperative complication in the late period of the hemorrhoidectomy is delayed wound healing. Hemorrhoid operation wound should be completely healed 6–8 weeks after the surgery. Incidence is 1–3%, and the main cause is from excessive excision of the anal mucosa [51, 52]. The symptoms are mucus discharge or small bleeding and stinging pain. Prevention would be the best treatment, but once occurred, the treatment should be based on the fissure treatment. Granulation tissue can be cauterized with using $AgNO_3$ and administer fiber. In the case of increased anal pressure, partial internal sphincterotomy can be performed in parallel on the opposite side. Excessive excision during surgery may cause anal stenosis. Anal stenosis usually occurs in patients with delayed wound healing, but it can also occur in patients without the pattern of the delayed wound healing (Fig. 5.8). Once the stenosis occurs, it has to be solved with sphincterotomy or advancement flap. But if sphincterotomy has risk of incontinence, advancement flap should be performed. And after the advancement flap, fiber should be administered.

5.7 Operative Treatment in Special Cases

Thrombotic external hemorrhoid can occur after diarrhea or constipation, excessive straining, or with sitting on toilet for long, but it can also occur without any specific factor (Fig. 5.9) [53]. It is easily diagnosed visually by round- or oval-shaped dark brown lump, and 48 hours after the occurrence, the pain reduces, and it can be treated with warm sitz bath and painkiller or stool softener. But in the case of severe pain, excisional operation should be performed immediately. Surgical excision is known for fast

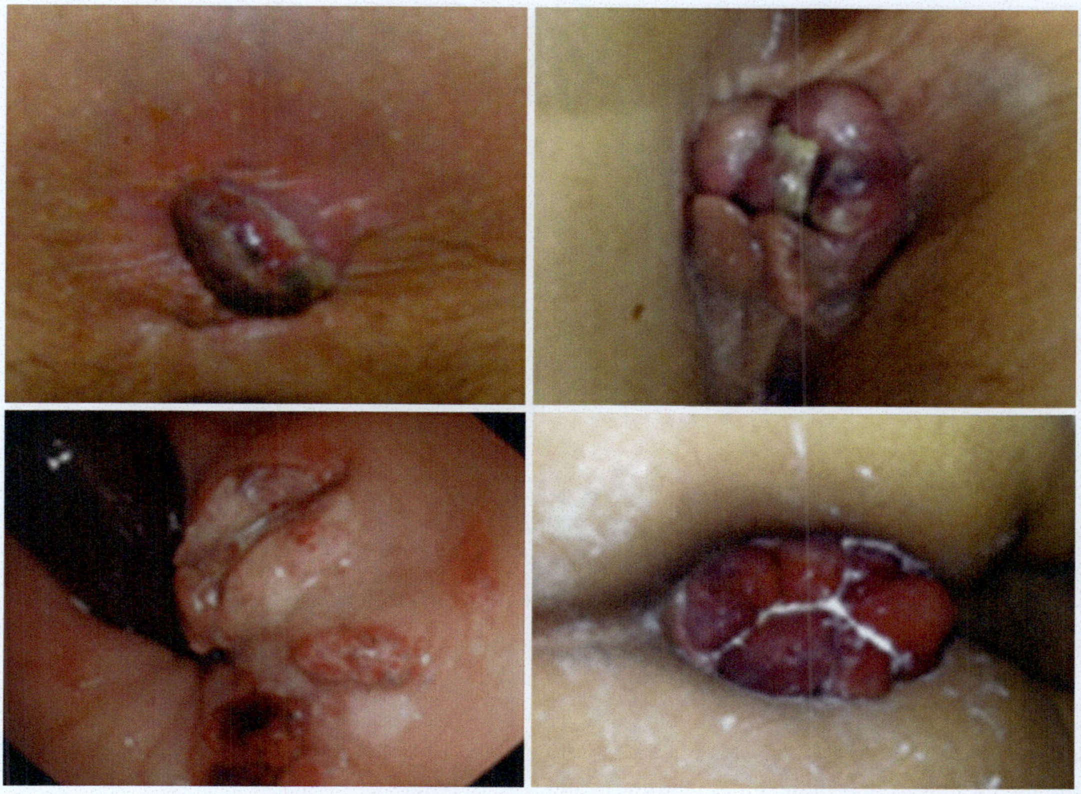

Fig. 5.9 Thrombotic external hemorrhoids

recovery and lower recurrence than the conservative treatment [54].

Thrombotic internal hemorrhoids can occur by leaving prolapsed hemorrhoids untreated and followed by blood circulation disorder. In the case of mild to moderate pain, therefore, symptoms can be treated with warm sitz bath. In the case of incarcerated circumferential thrombotic hemorrhoids that occurred in the anus, it is accompanied by severe pain, secretion, and edema with discomfort and should be operated immediately (Fig. 5.10). Main hemorrhoidal piles should be removed, and the thrombus should be removed only by dissecting submucosal space through the excised main wound not to make postoperative stenosis. Be cautious not to cause injury of the internal sphincter or excessive excision of the anal mucosa during operation as edema is severe. If the operation is performed when the edema has reduced following hospitalized and under pain management with warm sitz bath for a couple of days, the incidence of postoperative complications can be reduced.

In case of hemorrhoids with portal hypertension, the middle and inferior rectal vein circulates to the heart through the vena cava and does not cause severe bleeding during hemorrhoidectomy theoretically [55]. But when considering hemorrhoid operation, in the case of portal hypertension, it is mainly caused by liver cirrhosis and has high risk of bleeding due to low immunity and coagulation disorder; therefore, operation has to be carefully decided and performed after the improvement of hemostatic disorder. Do not excise all piles at once, but excise in 1- or 2-week interval. Hemorrhoids may get worse, or occur during pregnancy or after birth, but in general, the symptoms improve after birth. If there is prolapse 3 months after the birth or persistent bleeding after the conservative treatment, operation should be considered. And as incarcerated hemorrhoids accompanied by thrombosis have

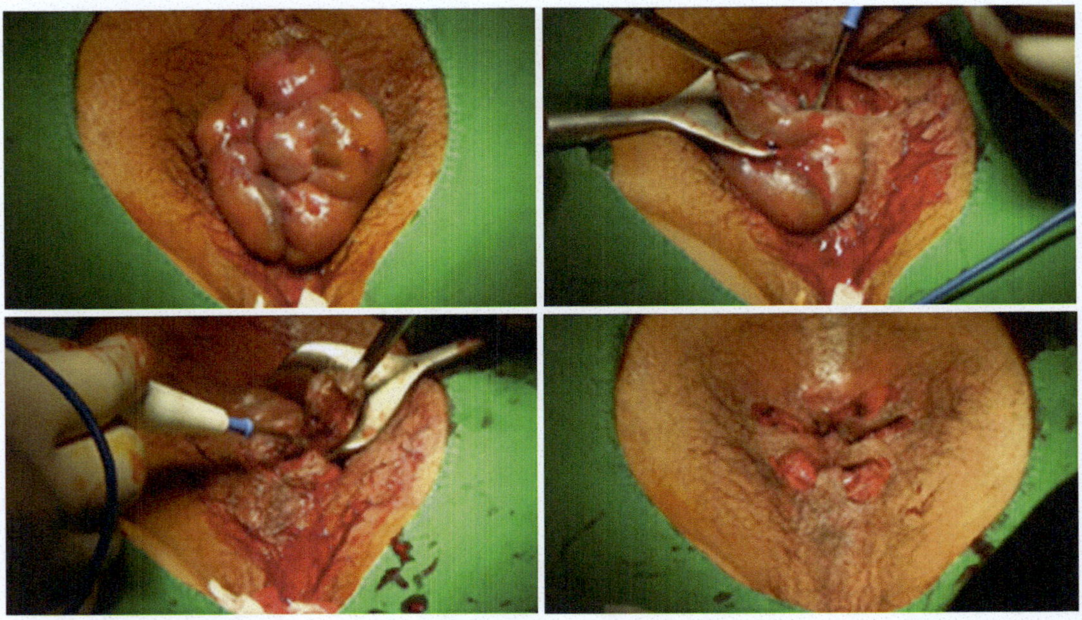

Fig. 5.10 Hemorrhoidectomy of Incarcerated or strangulated hemorrhoids

severe pain, operation is necessary. The operation should be performed under local anesthesia in lateral decubitus position, and severe hemorrhoidal piles causing symptoms should be selectively removed [56].

In ulcerative colitis or Crohn's disease, the hemorrhoids may occur or get worse by diarrhea, but if the diarrhea improves, the symptoms may improve. If the ulcerative colitis is in a stable status, operation can be performed selectively as the risk of postoperative complication is not so high. But in the case of Crohn's disease, the risk of postoperative complication is high, and wound healing is slow; therefore, it is a contraindication of the surgery [57, 58].

Immunocompromised patients with leukemia, lymphoma, and AIDS should avoid the operation and use conservative treatment, if it is not the case of strangulated thrombotic hemorrhoids, as the postoperative wound healing is difficult and easy to have abscess. If the operation is necessary, correct blood coagulation factor first, and use antibiotics prior to the operation [59].

5.8 Summary

The most common symptom in internal hemorrhoid is bleeding, and external hemorrhoid causes pain from stenosis. Doctors dealing with hemorrhoid should be well experienced with examination method and should be able to match appropriate examination method according to the patient's symptom. Most hemorrhoid symptoms can be improved with conservative treatment, but bleeding hemorrhoid can be effectively treated with rubber band ligation as it is hard to improve the symptoms. Excisional hemorrhoidectomy is best for prolapsed hemorrhoid or recurrent hemorrhoid treated with nonoperative treatment. The most common and discomforting postoperative complication is pain; therefore, pain management is important. Surgeon should be aware of the other postoperative complications and, especially, should be able to suspect inflammatory changes in the operated area if there's urinary retention or fever, and then the treatment should be performed immediately.

References

1. Thomson WHF. The nature of hemorrhoids. Br J Surg. 1975;62:542–52.
2. Haas PA, Fox TA Jr, Haas GP. The pathogenesis of hemorrhoids. Dis Colon Rectum. 1984;27:442–50.
3. Banov L, Knoepp LF, Erdman LH, Alia RT. Management of hemorrhoidal disease. J S C Med Assoc. 1985;81:398.
4. Harish K, Harikumar R, Sunilkumar K, Thomas V. Videoanoscopy: useful technique in the evaluation of hemorrhoids. J Gastroenterol Hepatol. 2008;23:e312–7.
5. Gralnek IM, Ron-Tal Fisher O, Holub JL, Eisen GM. The role of colonoscopy in evaluating hematochezia: a population-based study in a large consortium of endoscopy practices. Gastrointest Endosc. 2013;77:410–8.
6. Johannsson HO, Graf W, Pahlman L. Bowel habits in hemorrhoid patients and normal subjects. Am J Gastroenterol. 2005;100:401–6.
7. Garg P, Singh P. Adequate dietary fiber supplement along with TONE concept can helf avoid surgery in most patients with advanced hemorrhoids. Minerva Gastroenterol Dietol. 2017;63:92–6.
8. Alonso-Coello P, Zhou Q, Martinez-Zapata MJ, et al. Meta-analysis of flavonoids for the treatment of hemorrhoids. Br J Surg. 2006;93:909–20.
9. MacRae HM, McLeod RS. Comparison of hemorrhoidal treatment modalities: a meta-analysis. Dis Colon Rectum. 1995;38:687–94.
10. Law WL, Chu KW. Triple rubber band ligation for hemorrhoids: prospective, randomized trial of use of local anesthetic injection. Dis Colon Rectum. 1999;42(3):363–6.
11. Bayer I, Myslovaty B, Picovsky BM. Rubber band ligation of hemorrhoids. Convenient and economic treatment. J Clin Gastroenterol. 1996;23(1):50–2.
12. Khubchandani IT. A randomized comparison of single and multiple rubber band ligations. Dis Colon Rectum. 1983;26(11):705–8.
13. Iyer VS, Shrier I, Gordon PH. Long-term outcome of rubber band ligation for symptomatic primary and recurrent internal hemorrhoids. Dis Colon Rectum. 2004;47:1364–70.
14. El Nakeeb AM, Fikry AA, Omar WH, et al. Rubber band ligation for 750 cases of symptomatic hemorrhoids out of 2200cases. World J Gastroenterol. 2008;14:6525–30.
15. Khoury GA, Lake SP, Lewis MC, Lewis AA. A randomized trial to compare single with multiple phenol injection treatment for haemorrhoids. Br J Surg. 1985;72(9):741–2.
16. Yano T, Nogaki T, Asano M, Tanaka S, Kawakami K, Matsuda Y. Outcomes of case-matched injection sclerotherapy with a new agent for hemorrhoids in patients treated with or without blood thinners. Surg Today. 2013;43:854–8.
17. Miyamoto H, Hada T, Ishiyama G, Ono Y, Watanabe H. Aluminum potassium sulfate and tannic acid sclerotherapy for Goligher grades II and III hemorrhoids: results from a multi-center study. World J Hempatol. 2016;8:844–9.
18. Guy RJ, Seow-Choen F. Septic complications after treatment of haemorrhoids. Br J Surg. 2003;90:147–56.
19. Admi B, Eckardt VF, Suermann RB, Karbach U, Ewe K. Bacteremia after proctoscopy and hemorrhoidal injection sclerotherapy. Dis Colon Rectum. 1981;24:373–4.
20. Linares Santiago E, Gomez Parra M, Mendoza Olivares FJ, Pellicer Bautista FJ, Herrerias Gutierrez JM. Effectiveness of hemorrhoidal treatment by rubber band ligation and infrared photocoagulation. Rev Es Enferm Dig. 2001;93:238–47.
21. Ahmad A, Kant R, Gupta A. Comparative analysis of Doppler guided hemorrhoidal artery ligation (DG-HAL) & infrared coagulation (IRC) in management of hemorrhoids. Ind J Surg. 2013;75:274–72.
22. Ferguson JA, Mazier WP, Ganchrow MI, Friend WG. The closed technique of hemorrhoidectomy. Surgery. 1971;70(3):480–4.
23. Milligan ET, Morgan CN. Surgical anatomy of the anal canal and the operative treatment of hemorrhoids. Lancet. 1937;2:119–24.
24. Ruiz-Moreno F. Hemorrhoidectomy–how I do it: semiclosed technique. Dis Colon Rectum. 1977;20(3):177–82.
25. Ho YH, Seow-Choen F, Tan M, Leong AF. Randomized controlled trial of open and closed haemorrhoidectomy. Br J Surg. 1997;84(12):1729–30.
26. Gencosmanoglu R, Sad O, Koc D, Inceoglu R. Hemorrhoidectomy: open or closed technique? A prospective, randomized clinical trial. Dis Colon Rectum. 2002;45(1):70–5.
27. Bhatti MI, Sajid MS, Baig MK. Milligan-Morgan (open) versus Ferguson haemorrhoidectomy (closed): a systematic review and meta-analysis of published randomized, controlled trials. World J Surg. 2016;40:1509–19.
28. Xu L, Chen H, Lin G, Ge Q. Ligasure versus Ferguson hemorrhoidectomy in the treatment of hemorrhoids: a meta-analysis of randomized control trials. Surg Laparosc Endosc Percutan Tech. 2015;25:106–10.
29. Mushaya CD, Caleo PJ, Bartlett L, Buettner PG, Ho YH. Harmonic scalpel compared with conventional excisional haemorrhoidectomy: a meta-analysis of randomized controlled trials. Tech Coloproctol. 2014;18:1009–16.
30. Tsunoda A, Sada H, Sugimoto T, et al. Randomized controlled trial of bipolar diathermy vs ultrasonic scalpel for closed hemorrhoidectomy. World J Gastrointesti Surg. 2011;3:147–52.
31. Longo A. Treatment of haemorrhoidal disease by reduction for mucosa and haemorrhoidal prolapse with a circular stapling device: a new procedure-6th World Congress of Endoscopic Surgery. Mundozzi Editore. 1998. p. 777–84.

32. Lin HC, He QL, Ren DL, Peng H, Xie SK, Su D, et al. Partial stapled hemorrhoidopexy: a minimally invasive technique for hemorrhoids. Surg Today. 2012;42(9):868–75.
33. Lin HC, Ren DL, He QL, Peng H, Xie SK, Su D, et al. Partial stapled hemorrhoidopexy versus circular stapled hemorrhoidopexy for grade III-IV prolapsing hemorrhoids: a two-year prospective controlled study. Tech Coloproctol. 2012;16:337–43.
34. Jeong H, Hwang S, Ryu KO, Lim J, Kim HT, Yu HM, et al. Early experience with a partial stapled hemorrhoidopexy for treating patients with grades III-IV prolapsing hemorrhoids. Ann Coloproctol. 2017;33:28–34.
35. Shao WJ, Li GC, Zhang ZH, Yang BL, Sun GD, Chen YQ. Systematic review and meta-analysis of randomized controlled trials comparing stapled haemorrhoidopexy with conventional haemorrhoidectomy. Br J Surg. 2008;95(2):147–60.
36. Watson AJ, Hudson J, Wood J, Kilonzo M, Brown SR, McDonald A, Norrie J, Bruhn H, Cook JA, eTHoS Study Group. Comparison of stapled haemorrhoidopexy with traditional excisional surgery for haemorrhoidal disease (eTHoS): a pragmatic, multicentre, randomised controlled trial. Lancet. 2016;388:2375–85.
37. van Wensen RJ, van Leuken MH, Bosscha K. Pelvic sepsis after stapled hemorrhoidopexy. World J Gastroenterol. 2008;14(38):5924–6.
38. Faucheron JL, Voirin D, Abba J. Rectal perforation with life-threatening peritonitis following stapled haemorrhoidopexy. Br J Surg. 2012;99:746–53.
39. Aigner F, Bodner G, Gruber H, Conrad F, Fritsch H, Margreiter R, Bonatti H. The vascular nature of hemorrhoids. J Gastrointest Surg. 2006;10:1044–50.
40. Kalafateli M, Triantos CK, Nikolopoulou V, Burroughs A. Non-variceal gastrointestinal bleeding in patients with liver cirrhosis: a review. Dig Dis Sci. 2012;57:2743–54.
41. Emile SH, Youssef M, Elfeki H, Thabet W, El-Hamed TM, Farid M. Literature review of the role of lateral internal sphincterotomy (LIS) when combined with excisional hemorrhoidectomy. Int J Color Dis. 2016;31:1261–72.
42. Siddiqui MR, Abraham-Igwe C, Shangumanandan A, Grassi V, Swift I, Abulafi AM. A literature review on the role of chemical sphincterotomy after Milligan-Morgan hemorrhoidectomy. Int J Color Dis. 2011;26:685–92.
43. Gorfine SR, Onel E, Patou G, Krivokapic ZV. Bupivacaine extended-release liposome injection for prolonged postsurgical analgesia in patients undergoing hemorrhoidectomy: a multicenter, randomized, double-blind, placebo-controlled trial. Dis Colon Rectum. 2011;54:1552–9.
44. Haas E, Onel E, Miller H, Ragupathi M, White PF. A double-blind, randomized, active-controlled study for post-hemorrhoidectomy pain management with liposome bupivacaine, a novel local analgesic formulation. Am Surg. 2012;78:574–81.
45. Sugimoto T, Tsunoda A, Kano N, Kashiwagura Y, Hirose K, Sasaki T. A randomized, prospective, double-blind, placebo-controlled trial of the effect of diltiazem gel on pain after hemorrhoidectomy. World J Surg. 2013;37:2454–7.
46. Amoli HA, Notash AY, Shahandashti FJ, Kenari AY, Ashraf H. A randomized, prospective, double-blind, placebo-controlled trial of the effect of topical diltiazem on posthaemorrhoidectomy pain. Color Dis. 2011;13:328–32.
47. Liu JW, Lin CC, Kiu KT, Wang CY, Tam KW. Effect of glyceryl trinitrate ointment on pain control after hemorrhoidectomy: a meta-analysis of randomized controlled trials. World J Surg. 2016;40:215–24.
48. Wanis KN, Emmerton-Coughlin HM, Coughlin S, Foley N, Vinden C. Systemic metronidazole may not reduce posthemorrhoidectomy pain: a meta-analysis of randomized controlled trials. Dis Colon Rectum. 2017;60:446–55.
49. Vinson-Bonnet B, Higuero T, Faucheron JL, Senejoux A, Pigot F, Siproudhis L. Ambulatory haemorrhoidal surgery: systematic literature review and qualitative analysis. Int J Color Dis. 2015;30:437–45.
50. Toyonaga T, Matsushima M, Sogawa N, Jiang SF, Matsumura N, Shimojima Y, Tanaka Y, Suzuki K, Masuda J, Tanaka M. Postoperative urinary retention after surgery for benign anorectal disease: potential risk factors and strategy for prevention. Int J Color Dis. 2006;21:676–82.
51. Stelzner F. Hemorrhoidectomy–a simple operation? Incontinence, stenosis, fistula, infection and fatalities. Chirurg. 1992;63(4):316–26.
52. Sayfan J. Complications of Milligan-Morgan hemorrhoidectomy. Dig Surg. 2001;18(2):131–3.
53. Wronski K. Etiology of thrombosed external hemorrhoids. Postepy Hig Med Dosw (Online). 2012;66:41–4.
54. Greenspon J, Williams SB, Uoung HA, Orkin BA. Thrombosed external hemorrhoids. Outcome after conservative or surgical management. Dis Colon Rectum. 2004;47:1493–8.
55. Bernstein WC. What are hemorrhoids and what is their relationship to the portal venous system? Dis Colon Rectum. 1983;26:829–34.
56. Quijano CE, Abalos E. Conservative management of symptomatic and/or complicated haemorrhoids in pregnancy and the puerperium. Cochrane Database Syst Rev. 2005;(3):CD004077.
57. Cracco N, Zinicola R. Is haemorrhoidectomy in inflammatory bowel disease harmful? An old dogma re-examined. Color Dis. 2014;16:516–9.
58. D'Ugo S, Stasi E, Gaspari AL, Sileri P. Hemorrhoids and anal fissures in inflammatory bowel disease. Minerva Gastroenterol Dietol. 2015;61:223–33.
59. Morandi E, Merlini D, Salvaggio A, Foschi D, Trabucchi E. Prospective study of healing time after hemorrhoidectomy: influence of HIV infection, acquired immunodeficiency syndrome, and anal wound infection. Dis Colon Rectum. 1999;42:1140–4.

6 Anal Fissure

Sanghwa Yu

6.1 Introduction

Anal fissure is a longitudinal tear in squamous epithelium of the anal canal from anal verge up to the dentate line. It occurs mainly in posterior side, and about 10% occurs in anterior side of the anus which is more common in women. Main symptoms are severe tearing pain and a bright red blood on toilet paper, and with physical examination, laceration of the anal mucosa can be easily diagnosed. Patients often visit hospital if symptoms do not improve after weeks to months. Anal fissure is easily diagnosed by detail questioning and physical examination. In acute fissure, transverse fiber of the internal anal sphincter muscle or skin tags are not identified, but hypertrophied anal papilla is rare but can be found (Fig. 6.1) [1].

The margin of lacerated wound is fairly clean and hypertrophy is not identified. The duration of pain lasts from minutes to hours after defecation, and its severity varies greatly from person to person. Acute fissure untreated for longer than 6–8 weeks, the skin of lacerated wound swells and becomes bigger and repeats the symptom and makes fibrosis and hypertrophic skin tag (sentinel tag). As chronic mild inflammation repeats in lacerated wound, anal papilla occurs on the margin of the rectum from the fissure and gradually hypertrophied, followed by fibrosis, and grows bigger into a polyp shape, and at the fissure base, white internal sphincter is exposed (Fig. 6.2). But if the symptom is weakly repeated, even after 8 weeks, there could be no distinctive shape of the chronic fissure.

Sometimes, with severe chronic inflammation, it spreads through the sphincter and forms the intersphincteric abscess and ruptures to the skin and develops the intersphincteric anal fistula (Fig. 6.3).

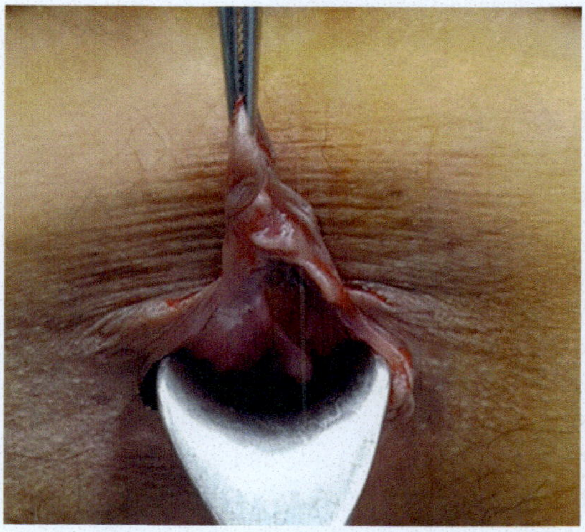

Fig. 6.1 Chronic anal fissure showing a hypertrophied anal papilla, sentinel pile (external skin tag), and exposed internal anal muscle fibers with raised edges

S. Yu (✉)
Colorectal Division, Department of Surgery, Hansol Hospital, Seoul, South Korea

D. K. Lee (ed.), *Practices of Anorectal Surgery*, https://doi.org/10.1007/978-981-13-1447-6_6

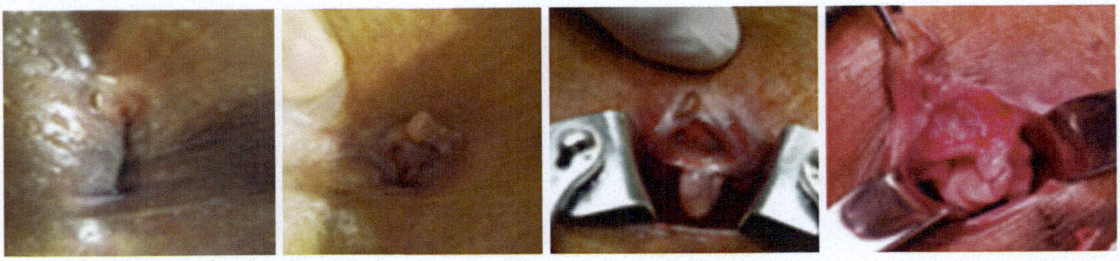

Fig. 6.2 From the acute phase to the chronic phase of the anal fissure

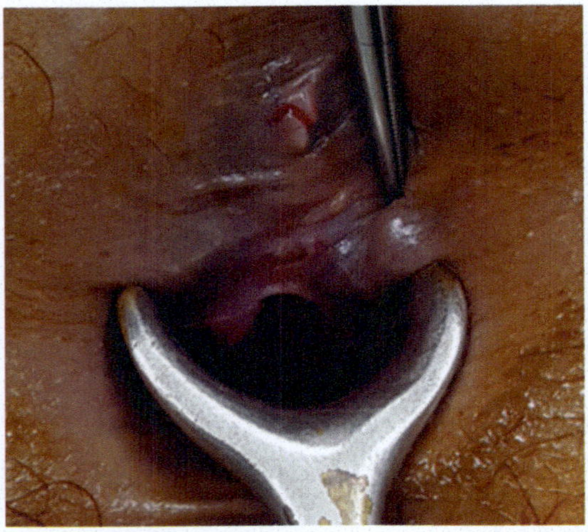

Fig. 6.3 Chronic anal fissure accompanied by intersphincteric anal fistula

6.2 Pathophysiology

It is not clear whether the tearing wound is the consequence of anal spasm or the anal spasm is the cause of tearing, but in general, the lacerated wound at the anal mucosa is occurred by an iatrogenic injury caused by hard stool. The pain from lacerated wound and the fear of pain cause tension in defecation, which causes internal sphincter spasm and hypertonia and increases the anal pressure and results in vicious circle and worsens the tearing. Most of the anal fissure (90%) occurs in posterior side of the anus as the skin is relatively inelastic and the blood flow in this area is relatively low [2, 3]. An anorectal angle by the puborectalis muscle tears easily by pressure in posterior midline in defecation. In anal fissure, the maximum resting pressure (MRP) is higher than the control group due to rectal distension which causes difficulty in relaxation of the internal sphincter, and ultra-slow wave is occasionally noticed, but it is reported that this wave disappears after the operation [4, 5]. High anal pressure decreases blood flow to the anal mucosa and causes ischemic change. Postmortem angiography presented by Klosterhalfen shows that hemorrhoidal artery has small branches in the internal anal sphincter, but in posterior midline, the branches are relatively less, and it is reported that ischemic change followed by the increase in anal pressure has great influence in this area [2]. Doppler flowmetry has shown an inverse relationship between the blood flow and MRP, and after the operation for the anal fissure, pressure dropped and blood circulation normalized. But it is not clear whether high anal resting pressure is the consequence or the cause of anal fissure.

Anterior anal fissure is observed in 10% of the patients and may have a different pathophysiology. It is mostly noticed in younger women and patients with injury or dysfunction of the external anal sphincter.

Atypical fissures (1%) – lateral or multiple fissures, fissures extending above the dentate line, and ulcerated fissure infiltrating into internal anal sphincter – are more likely to be the secondary fissure and through sufficient examinations should consider whether they are sexually transmitted diseases, leukemia, tuberculosis, Crohn's disease, or anal cancer [6].

6.3 Treatment

6.3.1 Conservative Treatment

Approximately 50% of patients with acute anal fissures can be treated with warm sitz bath, fiber intake, and stool softener [7]. It is most important to prevent damage in the anal mucosa from hard stool, and for this, sufficient amount of water and fiber should be taken. Pain from defecation increases the anal pressure from unconscious contraction, which is necessary for pain management. Warm sitz bath reduces pain by decreasing the anal pressure, and it is important in anal fissure treatment [8]. Because recurrence rate of anal fissure is fairly high, consistent fiber intake is recommended.

6.3.2 Non-operative Treatment

Only about 30% of chronic anal fissure is successful with conservative treatment, and this is because of internal sphincter hypertonia. Therefore, the treatment of chronic anal fissure should be combined with reducing internal sphincter hypertonia and conservative treatment. It is reported that approximately 50% of chronic fissure is successful with medical treatment, but this can differ depending on the duration, dosage, and number of medical treatment and on the patient's compliance. In medical treatment, consistent treatment is important, and if the treatment is stopped as symptoms disappear or the treatment is neglected from the first, it will not be cured. Once the treatment has started, it has to consist 2–3 months, and patients should be advised to improve lifestyle habits. Only 1/3 of chronic fissure is effective with conservative treatment, so other treatments should be considered and should target to treating to reduce the internal sphincter pressure.

6.3.2.1 0.2% Glyceryl Trinitrate (GTN) Ointment

Ever since the report of a nitric oxide or similar substances results in relaxation of internal sphincter, there have been a number of studies in adapting 0.2% glyceryl trinitrate (GTN) ointment to the patients with chronic anal fissure, and the success rate is about 50%. From the comparison studies of GTN treatment and control group, attentive effect has been observed in the improvement of the symptom and in the cure rate [9]. Even with increase of dosage, it did not respond to the treatment, and rather it increased the incidence of side effects [10, 11]. The most common side effect is headache, and more than 30% suffer from headache and 20% stop the treatment [12, 13]. Recurrence rate of GTN ointment is much higher than the operative treatment, and about half of the treated patients have recurrence [14]. If there's not respond to the treatment, that is to say, is recurred or stopped due to side effects, Botox injection or operative treatment should be considered.

6.3.2.2 Calcium Channel Blocker Ointment

Curative effect of calcium channel blocker (2% diltiazem or nifedipine) is similar to the GTN ointment, but headache side effect is less. It can be used for primary ointment treatment for chronic fissure [12, 13]; however, from some other research, it did not show better result than GTN [15, 16]. Topical ointment and oral medication have similar effect, but topical ointment is used, as it has less side effect like hypotension which can be seen in oral medication [17]. In comparative research among the Botox, the calcium channel blockers and diltiazem for chronic anal fissure, the cure rate after 3 months treatment was similar [18]. Similar to the GTN ointment, curative effect can be increased with constant use of the treatment.

6.3.2.3 Botox Injection

Botulinum toxin (type A) restrains acetylcholine secretion from the muscle and causes paralysis to reduce the anal pressure. The effect appears within the days and lasts for about 2–4 months. There is controversy on the dosage, method, and injection site, but in general, 20 U is injected into each side of fissure. It has less side effect compared to GTN or calcium channel blocker but can have temporary complications like flatus incontinence (18%) or fecal incontinence (5%), and the curative effect is reported to be 60~80% [7, 19]. Recurrence rate is somewhat high; however, it can be treated with repeat Botox injection and can have the similar curative effect as the previous treatment [20]. There have been a number of studies on GTN, calcium channel blocker, and Botox, and in general, Botox has better result than the topical ointment [21–23]. But as all the studies have been done with different dosage, method, and site, it is rather difficult to have constant result. In general case of chronic anal fissure, Botox can be used as secondary treatment failed from topical ointment, and for the patients with high risk of postoperative fecal incontinence (young and with birth injury women), it can be used prior to the operation [24, 25].

6.3.3 Operative Treatment

Anal ultrasound, anorectal physiology test, and common preoperative examinations like laboratory evaluation, chest X-ray, and EKG should be performed.

In general, surgery is performed under spinal anesthesia, but it can be performed under local anesthesia using epinephrine mixed lidocaine under intravenous sedation with propofol in case spinal anesthesia is difficult. In jack knife position, secure buttocks to the side of the surgery table using the tape and expose the anus.

6.3.3.1 Lateral Internal Sphincterotomy (Open or Close)

Digital anal dilatation (1984) is one of the initial forms of surgical treatment but no longer recommended as of high recurrence rate and risk of fecal incontinence [9]. There is a report that anal dilatation with balloon has lower risk of fecal incontinence and similar curative effect as lateral internal sphincterotomy, but the long-term result is unknown [26]. Eisenhammer's early sphincterotomy was performed on posterior side of the anus, and the result showed high incidence of fecal incontinence due to keyhole deformity. This was why Notaras performed slightly modified technique of lateral internal sphincterotomy, which reduced fecal incontinence complication and showed similar success rate. Surgical approach for chronic fissure was selected for the patient who failed from medical treatment. There are a few controversies on sphincterotomy, and one of them is whether to have open fashion or closed fashion. In closed fashion, insert scalpel and move forward to the dentate line and

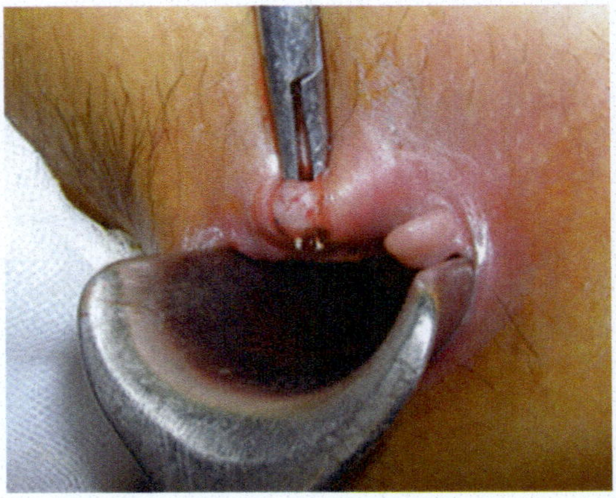

Fig. 6.4 Open lateral sphincterotomy

turn scalpel head to the anal mucosa, and having finger pressed down, cut internal sphincter relying on the sense. To prevent incomplete incision, press with finger to destroy remaining muscular fibers in internal sphincter after using scalpel. In open fashion, incise small anal verge, and in between the cut, use forceps to separate the internal sphincter with the anal mucosa and the external sphincter. Hold the incised internal sphincter with forceps, and use scalpel or scissor to incise up to the dentate line. Leave the incised skin open or sutured (Fig. 6.4). From many studies, the result of curative effect by the surgical method was similar [27–30], but open lateral internal sphincterotomy had higher complications and pain. Open technique can identify the cut range visually prior to incision; therefore, it is known to have less complications and high curative rate. Including us, in Korea, open technique is generally used. Another controversy is the incision range. With increase of the patients with postoperative complications like gas or fecal incontinence, Newstead and others reported that from the prospective study like tailored lateral sphincterotomy (incising as length of the fissure not from the dentate line), it showed similar recurrence rate but reduced the risk of incontinence [31–33]. The author also uses this technique and combines with conservative treatment to lower the surgery failure rate and complications. One of the main reasons that lateral internal sphincterotomy shows outstanding result compared to the medical treatment in chronic fissure is because patients tend to neglect the medical treatment. Even with high successful result, lateral internal sphincterotomy should be avoided in the patients with clear sphincter injury, history of anal surgery, inflammatory bowel disease, or birth injury.

6.3.3.2 Fissurectomy

By having the fissure base, margin and hypertrophied anal papilla, and skin tags excised all at once converts chronic fissure to acute fissure which induces healing. Be cautious as keyhole deformity can occur with having sphincterotomy performed at fissurectomy site. Fissurectomy is performed alone, but when combined with topical ointment or Botox, it is reported that the curative rate is higher (57.8–93%) [34, 35]. In some cases, to prevent sphincter spasm without the risk of fecal incontinence, fissurectomy site is covered with rectal mucosa or perianal skin (Fig. 6.5).

6.3.3.3 Advancement Flap

Advancement flap treats fissure by covering the fissure base with well-vascularized and healthy tissue. It is reported that in chronic fissure, anal pressure that is not too high can have high curative effect when combined with fissurectomy and can lower the risk of stenosis [36, 37]. In general, V-Y flaps are used, but sometimes island flap technique is also used. Unhealed fissure rate after advancement flap is 15–20%, and curative effect is lower than lateral internal sphincterotomy [38].

6.3.3.4 Anal Dilatation

Anal dilatation using finger or anal dilator is less effective than lateral internal sphincterotomy, and with high risk of permanent fecal incontinence, it is no longer recommended. However, nowadays, it is reported that cutting the internal sphincter muscle fibers with firm finger pressure or using dilators to slowly open the anus up to 48 mm in diameter or using pneumatic balloon result in similar effect as lateral internal sphincterotomy [39], but it is not performed in our clinic.

6.4 Treatment for Special Cases

In pregnancy period, one can have fissure due to constipation or hormonal change, but there is not much of an increased anal pressure. In acute phase, using conservative treatment such as stool softener or warm sitz bath can improve symptoms. But in chronic fissure, without incising internal sphincter, fissurectomy and advancement flap should be performed [40, 41].

In patients with Crohn's disease fissure occurs other than anterior or posterior part, in an atypical condition like deep ulcer and can accompany other anal diseases such as fistula. With proper medical treatment for Crohn's disease, over 50% of the anal diseases can be cured; therefore, surgical treatment should be avoided. However, if there is no respond to non-operative treatment and there is no other anorectal disease, surgical treatment can be considered on only selective patients (Fig. 6.6) [42, 43].

In the case of recurrence or unhealed fissure, through the anal ultrasound examination, check the result of lateral internal sphincterotomy. In case of incomplete sphincterotomy, additional sphincterotomy on the opposite side or advancement flap could be performed (Fig. 6.7).

Anal fissure in children is mostly related to constipation and encopresis, which can be treated with constipation treatment and warm sitz bath, and in most cases, symptoms disappear in 2 weeks. If there is no curative effect after 2-month treatment, topical ointment can be used as additional treatment, and surgical treatment is not considered.

6.5 Summary

Anal fissure accompanied by anal pain is a common anal disease; in the early stage, it can be treated by resolving sphincter hypertonia and softening the stool with conservative treatment. But fissure that does not respond to these treatments can be treated with topical ointment which reduces anal pressure by resolving sphincter hypertonia. However, if there is still no respond to

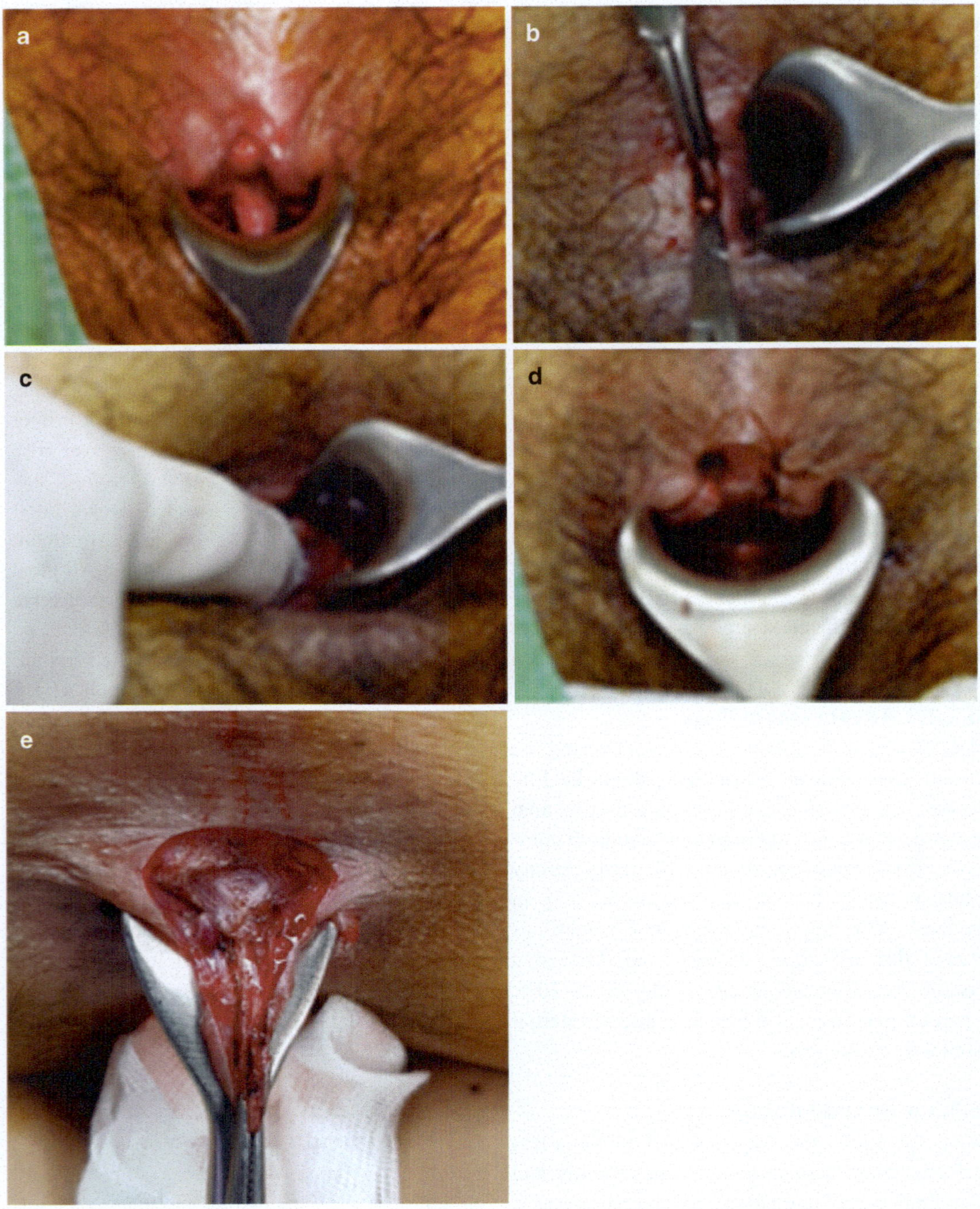

Fig. 6.5 Surgical procedure of open sphincterotomy for chronic anal fissure. (**a**) Chronic anal fissure with hypertrophic papilla. (**b**) Open lateral sphincterotomy. (**c**) Pressuring of the lateral side of the anal canal after sphincterotomy. (**d**) Marsupialization of edges of the fissurectomy wound. (**e**) Excision of the chronic anal fissure with hypertrophied papilla, and scar, and is left open

the treatment, Botox injection or surgery should be considered. The most common and safe surgical method is incising the internal sphincter, but as it has risk of fecal incontinence, nowadays, Botox or tailored sphincterotomy which is incising ulcer to the end is primarily performed. In the

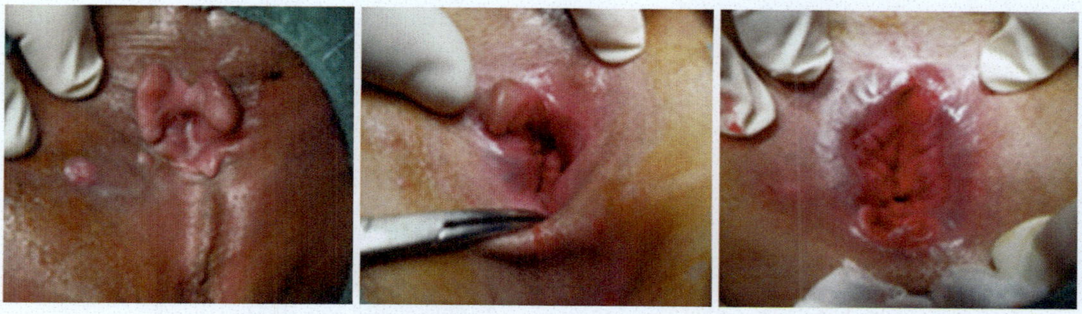

Fig. 6.6 Atypical features, such as multiple, large, lateral, or irregular fissures

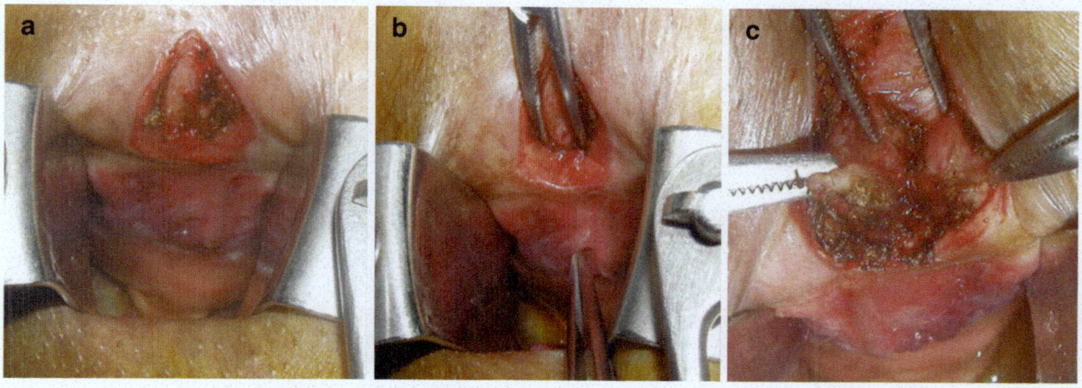

Fig. 6.7 Recurrent anal fissure. (**a**) Incomplete lateral sphincterotomy in the case of recurrence fissure. (**b**) Remained internal sphincter up to the dentate line. (**c**) Complete internal sphincterotomy

case of fissure that has no increase in anal pressure, fissurectomy and advancement flap surgery should be considered.

References

1. Clinical practice guideline for the management of anal fissures. Dis Colon Rectum. 2017;60:7–141.
2. Klosterhalfen B, Vogel P, Rixen H, Mittermayer C. Topography of the inferior rectal artery: a possible cause of chronic, primary anal fissure. Dis Colon Rectum. 1989;32(1):43–52.
3. Schouten WR, Briel JW, Auwerda JJ, De Graaf EJ. Ischaemic nature of anal fissure. Br J Surg. 1996;83:63–5.
4. Hancock BD. Measurement of anal pressure and motility. Gut. 1976;17:645–51.
5. Keck JO, Straniunas RJ, Coller JA, Barrett RC, Oster ME. Computer-generated profiles of the anal canal in patients with anal fissure. Dis Colon Rectum. 1995;38:72–9.
6. Lund JN, Scholefield JH. Aetiology and treatment of anal fissure. Br J Surg. 1996;83:1335–44.
7. Wald A, Bharucha AE, Cosman BC, Whitehead WE. ACG clinical guideline: management of benign anorectal disorders. Am J Gastroenterol. 2014;109:1141–57.
8. Gupta PJ. Randomized, controlled study comparing sitz-bath and no-sitz-bath treatments in patients with acute anal fissures. ANZ J Surg. 2006;76:718–21.
9. Nelson RL, Thomas K, Morgan J, et al. Non surgical therapy for anal fissure. Cochrane Database Syst Rev. 2012;(2):CD003431.
10. Altomare DF, Binda GA, Canuti S, Landolfi V, Trompetto M, Villani RD. The management of patients with primary chronic anal fissure: a position paper. Tech Coloproctol. 2011;15:135–41.
11. Scholefield JH, Bock JU, Marla B, Richter HJ, Athanasiadis S, Pröls M, Herold A. A dose finding study with 0.1%, 0.2%, and 0.4% glyceryl trinitrate ointment in patients with chronic anal fissures. Gut. 2003;52:264–9.
12. Ala S, Enayatifard R, Alvandipour M, Qobadighadikolaei R. Comparison of captopril (0.5%) cream with diltiazem (2%) cream for chronic anal fissure: a prospective randomized double-blind two-centre clinical trial. Color Dis. 2016;18:510–6.
13. Bailey HR, Beck DE, Billingham RP, Binderow SR, Gottesman L, Hull TL, Larach SW, Margolin

DA, Milsom JW, Potenti FM, Rafferty JF, Riff DS, Sands LR, Senagore A, Stamos MJ, Yee LF, Young-Fadok TM, Gibbons RD, Fissure Study Group. A study to determine the nitroglycerin ointment dose and dosing interval that best promote the healing of chronic anal fissures. Dis Colon Rectum. 2002;45:1192–9.
14. Berry SM, Barish CF, Bhandari R, Clark G, Collins GV, Howell J, Pappas JE, Riff DS, Safdi M, Yellowlees A. Nitroglycerin 0.4% ointment vs placebo in the treatment of pain resulting from chronic anal fissure: a randomized, double-blind, placebo-controlled study. BMC Gastroenterol. 2013;13:106.
15. Jonas M, Neal KR, Abercrombie JF, Scholefield JH. A randomized trial of oral vs. topical diltiazem for chronic anal fissures. Dis Colon Rectum. 2001;44:1074–8.
16. Sajid MS, Whitehouse PA, Sains P, Baig MK. Systematic review of the use of topical diltiazem compared with glyceryltrinitrate for the nonoperative management of chronic anal fissure. Color Dis. 2013;15:19–26.
17. Bulus H, Varol N, Tas A, Coskun A. Comparison of topical isosorbide mononitrate, topical diltiazem, and their combination in the treatment of chronic anal fissure. Asian J Surg. 2013;36:165–9.
18. Samim M, Twigt B, Stoker L, Pronk A. Topical diltiazem cream versus botulinum toxin a for the treatment of chronic anal fissure: a double-blind randomized clinical trial. Ann Surg. 2012;255:18–22.
19. Arroyo A, Perez F, Serrano P, et al. Long-term results of botulinum toxin for the treatment of chronic anal fissure: prospective clinical and manometric study. Int J Color Dis. 2005;20:267–71.
20. Nelson RL, Manuel D, Gumienny C, Spencer B, Patel K, Schmitt K, Castillo D, Bravo A, Yeboah-Sampong A. A systematic review and meta-analysis of the treatment of anal fissure. Tech Coloproctol. 2017;21:605–25.
21. Berkel AE, Rosman C, Koop R, van Duijvendijk P, van der Palen J, Klaase JM. Isosorbide dinitrate ointment vs botulinum toxin A (Dysport) as the primary treatment for chronic anal fissure: a randomized multicentre study. Color Dis. 2014;16:O360–6.
22. Sajid MS, Vijaynagar B, Desai M, Cheek E, Baig MK. Botulinum toxin vs glyceryl trinitrate for the medical management of chronic anal fissure: a meta-analysis. Color Dis. 2008;10:541–6.
23. Madalinski MH, Slawek J, Zbytek B, Duzynski W, Adrich Z, Jagiello K, Kryszewski A. Topical nitrates and the higher doses of botulinum toxin for chronic anal fissure. Hepato-Gastroenterology. 2001;48:977–9.
24. Lysy J, Israelit-Yatzkan Y, Sestiery-Ittah M, Weksler-Zangen S, Keret D, Goldin E. Topical nitrates potentiate the effect of botulinum toxin in the treatment of patients with refractory anal fissure. Gut. 2001;48:221–4.
25. Festen S, Gisbertz SS, van Schaagen F, Gerhards MF. Blinded randomized clinical trial of botulinum toxin versus isosorbide dinitrate ointment for treatment of anal fissure. Br J Surg. 2009;96:1393–9.
26. Renzi A, Izzo D, Di Sarno G, et al. Clinical, manometric, and ultrasonographic results of pneumatic balloon dilatation vs. lateral internal sphincterotomy for chronic anal fissure: a prospective, randomized, controlled trial. Dis Colon Rectum. 2008;51:121–7.
27. Nelson RL. Operative procedures for fissure in ano. Cochrane Database Syst Rev. 2010;(20):CD002199.
28. Boulos PB, Araujo JG. Adequate internal sphincterotomy for chronic anal fissure: subcutaneous or open technique? Br J Surg. 1984;71:360–2.
29. Kortbeek JB, Langevin JM, Khoo RE, Heine JA. Chronic fissure-in-ano: a randomized study comparing open and subcutaneous lateral internal sphincterotomy. Dis Colon Rectum. 1992;35:835–7.
30. Wiley M, Day P, Rieger N, Stephens J, Moore J. Open vs. closed lateral internal sphincterotomy for idiopathic fissure-in-ano: a prospective, randomized, controlled trial. Dis Colon Rectum. 2004;47:847–52.
31. Menteş BB, Ege B, Leventoglu S, Oguz M, Karadag A. Extent of lateral internal sphincterotomy: up to the dentate line or up to the fissure apex? Dis Colon Rectum. 2005;48:365–70.
32. Elsebae MM. A study of fecal incontinence in patients with chronic anal fissure: prospective, randomized, controlled trial of the extent of internal anal sphincter division during lateral sphincterotomy. World J Surg. 2007;31:2052–7.
33. Ho KS, Ho YH. Randomized clinical trial comparing oral nifedipine with lateral anal sphincterotomy and tailored sphincterotomy in the treatment of chronic anal fissure. Br J Surg. 2005;92:403–8.
34. Lindsey I, Cunningham C, Jones OM, Francis C, Mortensen NJ. Fissurectomy-botulinum toxin: a novel sphincter-sparing procedure for medically resistant chronic anal fissure. Dis Colon Rectum. 2004;47(11):1947–52.
35. Barnes TG, Zafrani Z, Abdelrazeq AS. Fissurectomy combined with high-dose botulinum toxin is a safe and effective treatment for chronic anal fissure and a promising alternative to surgical sphincterotomy. Dis Colon Rectum. 2015;58(10):967–73.
36. Patti R, Fama F, Tornambe A, Asaro G, Di Vita G. Fissurectomy combined with anoplasty and injection of botulinum toxin in treatment of anterior chronic anal fissure with hypertonia of internal anal sphincter: a pilot study. Tech Coloproctol. 2010;14(1):31–6.
37. Singh M, Sharma A, Gardiner A, Duthie GS. Early results of a rotational flap to treat chronic anal fissures. Int J Color Dis. 2005;20(4):339–42.
38. Leong AF, Seow-Choen F. Lateral sphincterotomy compared with anal advancement flap for chronic anal fissure. Dis Colon Rectum. 1995;38:69–71.
39. Renzi A, Izzo D, Di Sarno G, Talento P, Torelli F, Izzo G, Di Martino N. Clinical, manometric, and ultrasonographic results of pneumatic balloon dilatation vs. lateral internal sphincterotomy for chronic anal fissure: a prospective, randomized, controlled trial. Dis Colon Rectum. 2008;51:121–7.

40. Corby H, Donnelly VS, O'Herlihy C, O'Connell PR. Anal canal pressures are low in women with postpartum anal fissure. Br J Surg. 1997;84:86–8.
41. Patti R, Famà F, Barrera T, Migliore G, Di Vita G. Fissurectomy and anal advancement flap for anterior chronic anal fissure without hypertonia of the internal anal sphincter in females. Color Dis. 2010;12:1127–30.
42. Fleshner PR, Schoetz DJ Jr, Roberts PL, Murray JJ, Coller JA, Veidenheimer MC. Anal fissure in Crohn's disease: a plea for aggressive management. Dis Colon Rectum. 1995;38:1137–43.
43. Wolkomir AF, Luchtefeld MA. Surgery for symptomatic hemorrhoids and anal fissures in Crohn's disease. Dis Colon Rectum. 1993;36:545–7.

Anal Stenosis

7

Dong Woo Kang

7.1 Introduction

Anal stenosis refers to an abnormally narrowed anal canal. Due to etiology, anal canal transforms into a fibrous connective tissue losing its normal elasticity and hardening by fibrosis. In general, it occurs during cicatrization of the anal mucosa, and it can be limited to specific area or the entire anal canal. Khubchandani classified anal stenosis into congenital, primary, and secondary stenosis, and this classification is most widely used [1]. Congenital stenosis is the case of imperforated or anal developmental anomaly, and primary stenosis is a senile change or menopausal stenosis. Secondary stenosis is caused by postoperative stenosis, inflammatory disease such as Crohn's disease or tuberculosis, radiation exposure, and chronic use of laxatives [2]. In this chapter, we will focus on postoperative stenosis.

7.2 Etiology

There is difference in the incidence of anal stenosis patients by etiology, level of the hospital, and range of diseases dealt. In special hospital of the colorectal disease, 90% of anal stenosis is caused by postoperative stenosis from hemorrhoidectomy, due to excessive excision [3–5]. Anal stenosis can be followed by stapled hemorrhoidectomy [6] and inflammation by anastomotic disruption from anterior resection for rectal cancer, which mainly occurs in the upper side of the dentate line [7]. Anal stenosis caused by inflammatory bowel disease, especially stenosis due to Crohn's disease, is increasing. Stenosis from Crohn's disease is due to transmural scarring of inflammatory process, and recurrence is common and usually does not respond to surgery, which can result in permanent enterostomy [8]. If a laxative is used daily for a long period, it results in anal stenosis from gradual and irreversible fibrosis of the submucosal layer due to loss of normal dilation of the anus during bowel movement [9].

7.3 Classification

Milsom and Mazier classified anal stenosis by range, mild (tight anal canal for the medium Hill-Ferguson retractor and lubricated index finger), moderate (forceful dilatation required for the retractor and index finger), and severe (difficult even for small retractor or little finger), and also classified stenosis by site: low (up to 0.5 cm below the dentate line from the anal verge), middle (0.5 cm below the dentate line to the 0.5 cm upper dentate line), and high (from the 0.5 cm upper dentate line and up) [2].

D. W. Kang (✉)
Colorectal Division, Department of Surgery, Hansol Hospital, Seoul, South Korea
e-mail: kdw@hansolh.co.kr

D. K. Lee (ed.), *Practices of Anorectal Surgery*, https://doi.org/10.1007/978-981-13-1447-6_7

7.4 Diagnosis

The most common symptoms are defecation difficulty and anal pain. Especially after hemorrhoidectomy, the pain is severe due to poor healing. Other symptoms are constipation and tenesmus, and in severe cases, stenosis worsens with anal damage and bleeding caused by finger used to dig out the stool. Also, diarrhea due to long-term use of laxative and watery stool from fecal impaction occur. Over time, outlet obstructive constipation due to stenosis dilates the rectum and causes megarectum [7].

Diagnosis of an anal stenosis is easily done with digital anal examination, and through detailed history taking, the cause of stenosis can be determined, and the degree of stenosis can be checked through physical examination. Sometimes it is necessary to identify the site of stenosis by evaluation under anesthesia, and this makes it possible to check for lesion of rectal mucosa using proctoscopy, and biopsy can be performed to determine other diseases [9]. If there is eczematoid or ulcerative lesion, it is necessary to differentiate for Bowen's disease or Paget's disease. Also, it needs to be distinguished for anal cancer, wart lesion, and STD (sexually transmitted disease) through the anus. Stenosis with cicatrization from past surgery usually has smooth form with loss of elasticity. If not, additional examination may be needed for diagnosis, or biopsy may be necessary. It is useful to have anal manometry among anal physiology tests and measure anal sphincter pressure, rectal compliance, and recto-anal inhibitory reflex which can help to determine treatment plan and evaluate anal function. Anal ultrasound, however, does not help to determine the treatment plan or diagnosis of stenosis, and it is generally not performed, as ultrasonic instrument is difficult to enter the narrowed anal canal.

7.5 Treatment

The best treatment for anal stenosis is prevention. Delicate and adequate anorectal surgery can reduce incidence of stenosis. Prevent excessive excision of the anal mucosa, and maintain adequate mucosal bridge between the wounds, and it is important to use absorbable suture thread.

7.5.1 Conservative Treatment

In mild or moderate anal stenosis, sufficient fluid supply and bulking agent such as stool softeners and fiber supplements help the anal canal to dilate naturally for a smooth bowel movement and bulky stool [10]. It is very effective if constant dilatation can be performed with dilator or fingertip with sufficient amount of lubricant, but due to pain, it is not easy (Fig. 7.1) [3]. Anal dilatation also can cause mucosal damage or hematoma in the anal muscular layer, and should be cautious not to progress stenosis by fibrosis.

The dilator is gently inserted into the anus with lubrication. Dilatation will continue until the anus has reached the desired size.

7.5.2 Operative Treatment

Lateral internal sphincterotomy is recommended for the patients with mild stenosis or unresolved fissure after hemorrhoidectomy. At this time,

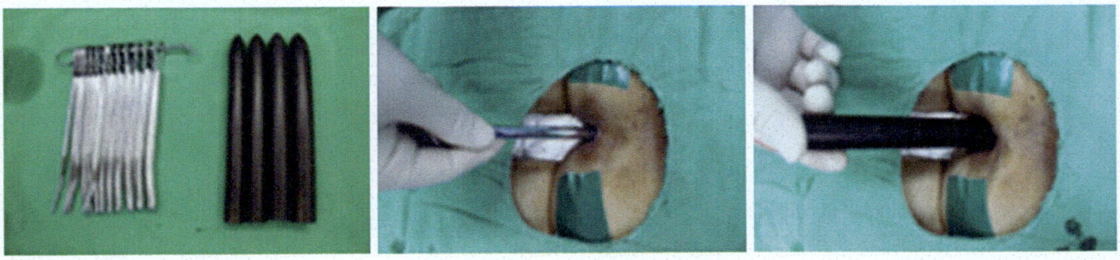

Fig. 7.1 Hegar's dilators

longitudinal incision should be performed on scarred area to have anal dilate appropriately. Incision wound should be left for secondary healing. Bulking agents such as fiber or stool softener should be used for long period of time to prevent recurrence after the operation [3]. Prior to the operation, functional test including anal manometry should be performed to exclude patients with high risk of fecal incontinence after sphincterotomy. Moderate or severe stenosis is considered for surgical treatment to replace the inelastic anal mucosa with new elastic anal mucosa. In this case, if the cicatricial fibrosis is accompanied, sphincterotomy should be combined with advancement flap. Advancement flap or rotational S-flap is the typical surgical methods, and colorectal surgeons should be well skilled and experienced. The design of the flap is very important as the blood supply to transposition or advancement flap is supplied directly from small vessel below the flap, when the blood supplies to the rotational S-flap is supplied from the named vessel [11, 12].

A surgical method should be determined under the preference of the surgeon and range, degree, and site of stenosis. For moderate stenosis, Y-V advancement flap, V-Y advancement flap, rhomboid-shaped or diamond-shaped advancement flap is mainly used, and for high-level stenosis, house flap is mainly used (Fig. 7.2) [13–15].

For severe stenosis, it can be resolved with flapping on both sides. Rotational S-flap is rarely used, except for stenosis after Paget's disease or Bowen's disease surgery.

Bowel preparation is usually needed prior to the surgery. Second-generation cephalosporin and metronidazole are intravenously injected just before the operation for the prevention of infection. The operation is performed in prone jackknife position under spinal anesthesia (Fig. 7.3) [14, 16].

Stage 1: After evaluating the degree of anal stenosis, lone star retractor is installed. Retractor should be installed on each anterior and posterior side. Design flap shape with a pen on the side of a healthy anal skin. The size of the flap should be about 15 mm in each side, and the base of the flap should be able to move up to the stenosis.

Stage 2: Incision is performed with scalpel from the base of the flap to the proximal of stenosis.

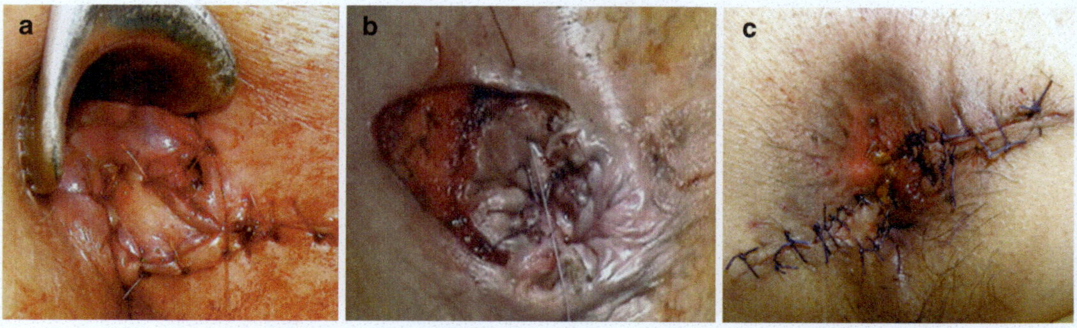

Fig. 7.2 Anoplasty with various types of flaps. (**a**) House-shaped flap. (**b**) V-Y advancement flap. (**c**) Bilateral House-shaped flap

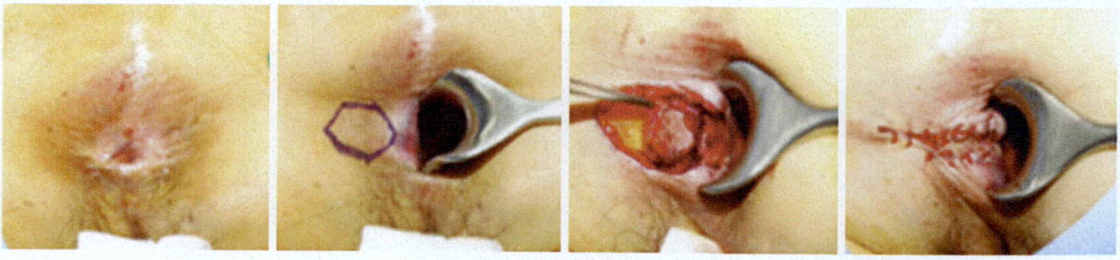

Fig. 7.3 Diamond flap for anal stenosis

To prevent postoperative fecal incontinence, incise partial internal sphincter up to 25 mm caliber of the anus. Following each side of the flap, incise the subcutaneous fat layer, undermining along each side leaving sufficient pedicle part on the center below the flap, which facilitates movement.

Stage 3: After removing the installed retractor, simple mattress suture by 2~3 mm intervals using 4-0 vicryl suture on each side of the transferred flap. Be cautious not to cause flap ischemia from excessive suture tension. And simple mattress suture using 4-0 vicryl suture on the original flap sides, but the end part is left open for drainage.

7.5.2.1 Mucosal Advancement Anoplasty

It is performed in prone jack-knife position under local or spinal anesthesia after bowel preparation. Scar tissue is removed by vertical incision from the anal verge to the dentate line. Undermine about 2~5 cm below the rectal mucosa, and pull down for interrupted suture at the end of internal sphincter, and leave the outer wound open. Be cautious not to cause seepage of the mucus by suturing too far below (Fig. 7.4) [17, 18].

7.5.2.2 Y-V Anoplasty

Y shape is formed from incising narrowed anal mucosa and V-shaped incision on the outer side. Undermine at least 2 cm of perianal skin and pull into anal canal and suture in V shape. It can be used for posterior or lateral stenosis but is generally used for the stenosis under the dentate line, as it has limit in the movement of the flap (Fig. 7.5) [19–22].

Fig. 7.4 Mucosal advancement flap

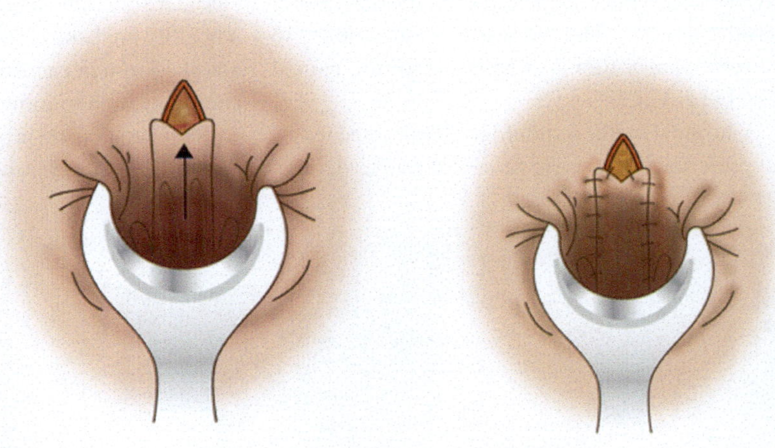

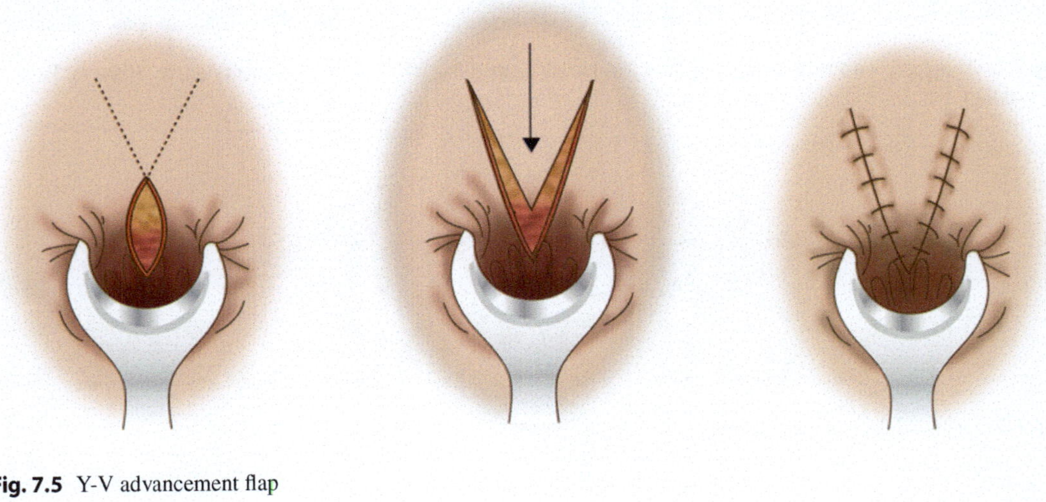

Fig. 7.5 Y-V advancement flap

7.6 Postoperative Management and Complications

Postoperative management should be followed on the next day of the operation by warm sitz bath, and administer fiber supplement. Antibiotics should be administered for 3 days after injecting once the intravenous injection. Stool softener is not used as diarrhea can worsen the wound. When S-flap plasty or bilateral flap surgery is performed, use antidiarrheal agents for 5 days to control bowel movement, and then warm sitz bath and fiber should be administered. Surgical treatment of anal stenosis can lead to various complications. Necrosis of the flap, wound infection, suture failure, and other problems may occur, followed by failure of stenosis correction, restenosis due to ischemic contraction, and fecal incontinence. Therefore, delicate surgery is essential by experienced surgeon.

7.7 Summary

Although anal stenosis is a rare complication, but once it occurs, it is difficult to resolve. The most common cause of stenosis is hemorrhoidectomy, and as prevention is the best treatment, you should prevent excessive excision of the anal mucosa during surgery. If it cannot be treated with conservative treatment, then advancement flap surgery is the most effective surgical option.

References

1. Khubchandani IT. Anal stenosis. Surg Clin N Am. 1994;74(6):1353–60.
2. Milsom J, Mazier W. Classification and management of postsurgical anal stenosis. Surg Gynecol Obstet. 1986;163(1):60–4.
3. Liberman H, Thorson AG. How I do it. Anal stenosis. Am J Surg. 2000;179(4):325–9.
4. Puia IC, Bodea R, Neagoe RM. Hemorrhoidectomy and anal stenosis. J Gastrointestin Liver Dis. 2015;24:395–6.
5. Brisinda G. How to treat haemorrhoids: prevention is best; haemorrhoidectomy needs skilled operators. BMJ. 2000;321:582–3.
6. Wilson MS, Pope V, Doran HE, Fearn SJ, Brough WA. Objective comparison of stapled anopexy and open hemorrhoidectomy: a randomized, controlled trial. Dis Colon Rectum. 2002;45:1437–44.
7. Katdare MV, Ricciardi R. Anal stenosis. Surg Clin North Am. 2010;90:137–45.
8. Brochard C, Siproudhis L, Wallenhorst T, Cuen D, d'Halluin PN, Garros A, Bretagne JF, Bouguen G. Anorectal stricture in 102 patients with Crohn's disease: natural history in the era of biologics. Aliment Pharmacol Ther. 2014;40(7):796–803.
9. Shawki S, Costedio M. Anal fissure and stenosis. Gastroenterol Clin N Am. 2013;42:729–58.
10. Bristinda G, Vanella S, Cadeddu F, Marniga G, Mazzeo P, Brandara F, et al. Surgical treatment of anal stenosis. World J Gastroenterol: WJG. 2009;15(16):1921.
11. Duieb Z, Appu S, Hung K, Nguyen H. Anal stenosis: use of an algorithm to provide a tension-free anoplasty. ANZ J Surg. 2010;80:337–40.
12. Asfar S. Anoplasty for post-hemorrhoidectomy low anal stenosis: a new technique. World J Surg. 2018 Sep;42(9):3015–20.
13. Eu KW, Teoh TA, Seow-Choen F, Goh HS. Anal stricture following haemorrhoidectomy: early diagnosis and treatment. Aust N Z J Surg. 1995;65:101–3.
14. Gülen M, Leventoğlu S, Ege B, Menteş BB. Surgical treatment of anal stenosis with diamond flap anoplasty performed in a calibrated fashion. Dis Colon Rectum. 2016;59(3):230–5.
15. Farid M, Youssef M, El Nakeeb A, Fikry A, El Awady S, Morshed M. Comparative study of the house advancement flap, rhomboid flap, and y-v anoplasty in treatment of anal stenosis: a prospective randomized study. Dis Colon Rectum. 2010;53(5):790–7.
16. Sloane J, Zahid A, Young C. Rhomboid-shaped advancement flap anoplasty to treat anal stenosis. Tech Coloproctol. 2017;21(2):159–61.
17. Casadesus D, Villasana LE, Diaz H, et al. Treatment of anal stenosis: a 5-year review. ANZ J Surg. 2007;77:557–9.
18. Rakhmanine M, Rosen L, Khubchandani I, Stasik J, Riether R. Lateral mucosal advancement anoplasty for anal stricture. BJS. 2002;89:1423–4.
19. Maria G, Brisinda G, Civello IM. Anoplasty for the treatment of anal stenosis. Am J Surg. 1998;175:158–60.
20. Angelchik PD, Harms BA, Starling JR. Repair of anal stricture and mucosal ectropion with YV or pedicle flap anoplasty. Am J Surg. 1993;166:55–9.
21. Aitola P, Hiltunen K, Matikainen M. YV anoplasty combined with internal sphincterotomy for stenosis of the anal canal. Eur J Surg Acta Chir. 1997;163:839–42.
22. Gingold B, Arvanitis M. YV anoplasty for treatment of anal stricture. Surg Gynecol Obstet. 1986;162:241–2.

8 Perianal Abscess

Seung Han Kim

8.1 Introduction

It is essential in the treatment of perianal abscess to understand the relation between the anal sphincter and the spaces formed by the levator muscle.

8.2 Pathophysiology

Ninety percent of anorectal abscess is from the anal gland origin inflammation in the dentate line, blocked with feces or foreign body followed by the drainage difficulties. Inflammation from the anal gland infection is the primary focus, and an abscess is formed from the spread of inflammation to the surrounding spaces [1–4]. Other special cases which cause abscess around the anus would be tuberculosis, ulcerative colitis, Crohn's disease, and cancer. Especially 10–20% of Crohn's disease patients have anorectal abscess or anal fistula, and the incidence is much higher in the specialized hospitals [5–7]. As it is not a general anal gland infection but rather it occurs from the inflammation diseases that penetrate muscular walls, the treatment approach should be different from the general perianal abscess or fistula [8]. There are also rare cases like inflammation caused from the invaded bacteria where anal fissure occurred, suppurated inflammation from rupture of thrombosed external hemorrhoid, abscess from prolapsed internal hemorrhoid infection, abscess formed from postoperative local anesthesia in perianal area, and infection on the wound caused from bowel enema. It is mostly seen in the age of 20 to 40 in men.

8.3 Classification

Anorectal abscess is classified by the surrounding area of anal sphincter (Fig. 8.1) [4, 9, 10].

8.3.1 Perianal or Subcutaneous Abscess

Perianal subepithelial or perianal subcutaneous abscess is a very common abscess having inflammation spread in the subcutaneous fat layer from intersphincteric space.

8.3.2 Intersphincteric Abscess

Inflammation from the intersphincteric space near the dentate line coming down toward the anal verge is called the low type, and from here spreading to the rectum is called the high type. The low type especially causes severe pain in defecating and swelling near the anus and is

S. H. Kim (✉)
Colorectal Division, Department of Surgery, Hansol Hospital, Seoul, South Korea

D. K. Lee (ed.), *Practices of Anorectal Surgery*, https://doi.org/10.1007/978-981-13-1447-6_8

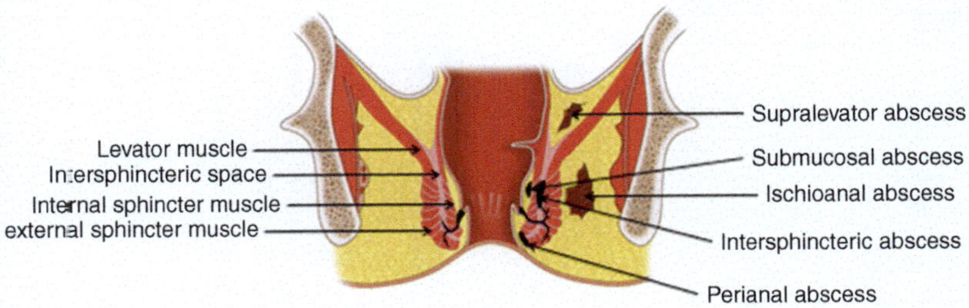

Fig. 8.1 Classification of anorectal suppuration

easy to diagnose as it has severe local tenderness on pressure. The high type which is stagnated in the rectum above the dentate line starts with heavy feeling and pain worsened with edema palpated from the digital examination, and it is necessary to distinguish from the submucosa abscess.

8.3.3 Ischiorectal Abscess

Ischiorectal abscess refers to the abscess stagnated in the ischiorectal space. In general, it starts from the inflammation at intersphincteric space and spreads through the external sphincter. It penetrates the external sphincter from posterior side of the anus and stagnates in the deep or superficial postanal space. Especially, the deep postanal space abscess forms a horseshoe abscess by spreading out to the lateral side of the ischiorectal fossa.

8.3.4 Supralevator Abscess

Abscess that occurs in the space between the rectum and the levator muscle and the incidence is not high. In most of the cases, inflammation occurs in the anal crypt of intersphincteric space near the dentate line and spreads upward and forms an abscess in the supralevator space. In rare cases, it spreads from intraperitoneal inflammation like diverticulitis of the colon, ulcerative colitis, and Crohn's disease. In some cases, it can occur from penetrated levator muscle from ischiorectal abscess, but it seems to occur from a mistakenly penetrated levator muscle when draining the ischiorectal fossa abscess [2–5].

8.4 Diagnosis

8.4.1 Examination

Anal pain is the most common symptom and easy to distinguish from fissure or thrombosed pain. Initially, there is no correlation with bowel movement, but over time, patients suffer from defecation disorders and pain during defecation and then gradually become feverish, and the pain becomes worse.

Through the digital anal examination, you can identify erythema and swelling in the perianal area and can feel the lump by pressing the side of skin with thumb and index finger in the anus, and patients suffer from the tenderness on pressure. In the case with superficial abscess, it is easy to identify erythema and swelling, but in the cases with ischiorectal fossa or deep postanal space or pelvirectal abscess, there is almost no erythema or swelling. In this case, patients suffer from generalized weakness and migrant fever, and it can be misdiagnosed as cold and flu. Through digital examination, you can feel a big thick lump in the posterolateral side of the lower rectum and anal canal including puborectalis, and as there's tenderness on pressure, it is easy to be diagnosed by the experienced doctor with digital examination. High intersphincteric abscess is also diagnosed by digital examination, and from the upper anal canal, you can identify the soft diffuse induration with tenderness on pressure. Most of the anorectal abscess can be diagnosed by the patient's symptom and physical examination in the outpatient clinic, but to distinguish from other diseases, it is sometimes examined under anesthesia. And in some cases, through anoscopy, you can identify the abscess from anal crypt.

8.4.2 Imaging Studies

Most of the anorectal abscess can be diagnosed without help of imaging studies, but in the cases with supralevator abscess or recurrent abscess or occur with other complex diseases, it may need imaging studies. Transanal ultrasonography is the most commonly used examination, and it can identify the presence and the range of abscess, but it is limited in examining supralevator space or outside of the external sphincter. Also, it has negative side, as it can cause pain by inserting ultrasonic device into anal canal and relies on the ability of the clinician [11]. Transperineal sonography has less pain, and it is an effective diagnostic tool, but it is limited in diagnosing the high-type abscess like perirectal abscess [12]. There is controversy on the usability of CT; it can be performed in cases with uncertainty of abscess from the physical examination or when suspecting supralevator abscess, and it can identify the stagnated abscess or air shadow [13]. Through MRI, you can have more precise information of the range of abscess and anatomical relation compared to the CT or ultrasound, and as it can be performed without pain, it is useful for complex abscess or recurrent abscess; the only negative side would be the high expense [14].

8.5 Treatment

8.5.1 Incision and Drainage

Prompt incision and drainage is most important, and for the incision of abscess, incise from near the anal verge and a small excision on the skin of the incision site to make a drainage hole in oval shape (Fig. 8.2). In the cases of superficial abscess, incision and drainage can be done under lidocaine local anesthesia, but for an exact assess of the abscess range and appropriate drainage, it is more comfortable for both doctors and patients to have it performed under spinal anesthesia. After the incision and drainage, insert finger and check for undrained abscess due to lattice formation in the anal space. Antibiotics are only used in immunocompromised patient, no improvement

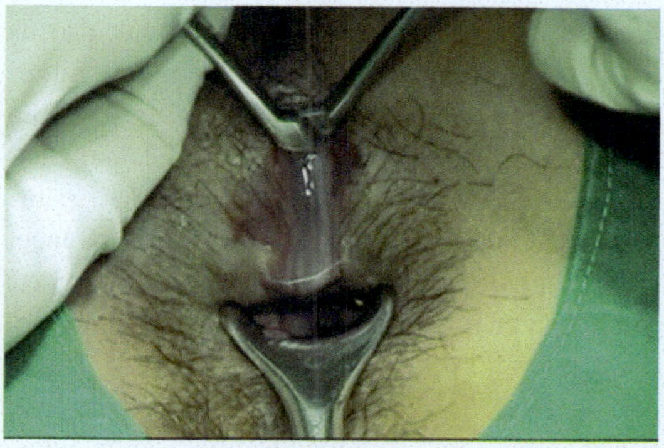

Fig. 8.2 Incision and drainage of perianal abscess (6 o'clock direction)

after drainage, accompanied with cellulitis, or diabetics [15, 16]. Bacteria culture test should be performed in the high-risk patients or in recurrent or those with persistent abscess. The fundamental principle of incision and drainage is to drain the abscess that penetrated the external sphincter toward the perianal skin and other abscess toward the rectum or anal canal. Deep postanal abscess is drained from the outside of the sphincter or intersphincteric approach [17], but in the case of simple incision and drainage, it is better to perform intersphincteric approach as it has less damage in the sphincter. In a wide range of abscess, catheter is inserted for drainage but we prefer to apply seton.

8.5.2 Incision and Drainage and Primary Fistulotomy

One of the most controversial in anal abscess treatment is whether to perform only simple incision and drainage or perform curative surgery on the anal fistula. The reason of the controversy is that some doctors claim that even with the simple incision and drainage, it can heal 60% of anal abscess without developing into anal fistula, and also in the case with abscess, due to edema and inflammation, it is likely to misplace the probe with incorrect internal opening or make wide surgical site or high risk in sphincter dysfunction. But other doctors have the concept that, unlike infant abscess, most of adult abscess develop into anal fistula, therefore it is recommended to combine curative surgery on the fistula and also as with the fistulotomy dysfunction from the sphincter damage is not so high [18–21]. Based on the 2010 Cochrane review, in the case of incision and drainage, by combining the fistulotomy or fistulectomy, you can reduce anal fistula recurrence, and eventually, it can reduce additional surgery. There can be a minimal damage to anal function, but there is no statistical significance [22]. If it is certain that the abscess is simple abscess like perianal abscess, submucous abscess or intersphincteric abscess and the inflammation started from the anal gland, then even with the primary fistulotomy, incontinence complication from the sphincter damage is minimal and could be the indication of incision and drainage and fistulotomy.

8.5.3 Drainage and Seton Application

In the anorectal abscess treatment, if there is concern of anal dysfunction due to incision and drainage and fistulotomy, then seton application can be an alternative treatment (Fig. 8.3). Seton application has smaller wound than fistulotomy with less postoperative pain and faster healing which makes it possible for persistent drainage. Also, with small wound, postoperative management is much simple and convenient. In cases of complex abscesses like ischiorectal abscess, deep postanal abscess, or supralevator abscess, it is difficult to drain with only simple incision and drainage, and also it could not be possible to drain persistently (Fig. 8.4). If the primary

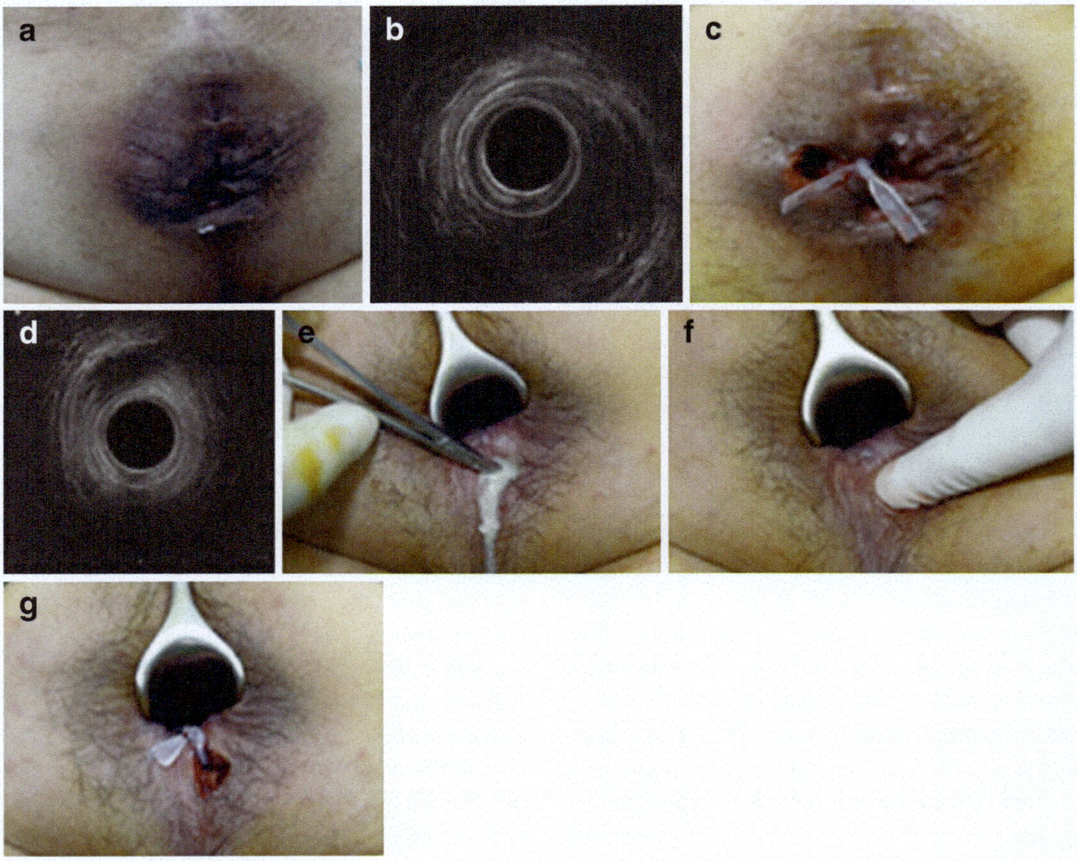

Fig. 8.3 Drainage and seton application for perianal abscess. (**a**) Erythematous swelling is seen at 5 o'clock. (**b**) Sonographic image of perianal abscess (5′). (**c**) Drainage of perianal abscess and seton application. (**d**) Sonographic image of perianal abscess (12 o'clock). (**e**) Incision and drainage of abscess. (**f**) Visible internal opening of perianal abscess. (**g**) Seton application

opening is certain, it is effective to apply drain seton and perform curative surgery afterwards [17, 22]. For complex abscess, even with certain primary opening, with fistulotomy there can be great sphincter damage and difficulty in wound management, and postoperative pain is severe. In the case of complex abscess with uncertain internal opening or no certainty in anatomical structure, it is better to finish the surgery with inserting drain tube after the incision and drainage (Fig. 8.5). Complex abscess is often misdiagnosed as cold and flu which delays the diagnosis of abscess. Deep postanal abscess is drained from posterior side of the external sphincter or drained from intersphincteric space after identifying the inflammatory site. In most cases, an internal opening is in the posterior side of the anal canal near the dentate line where the drain seton is applied. If the inflammation or abscess is spread to the lateral, then make a drainage hole in the lateral side, and apply each seton from the posterior to the lateral side; this is called modified Hanley's operation [23–26]. Supralevator abscess is drained into the rectum, so you can incise the rectal wall in the height of the spread inflammation from the dentate line, drain wound, and apply drain seton or drain after a complete incision of the rectal wall [14]. Sufficient hemostasis is essential as the rectal incision can cause bleeding.

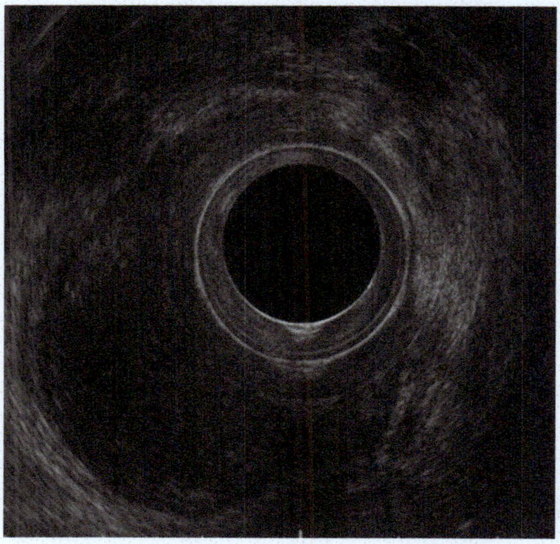

Fig. 8.4 Large hypoechoic lesion at 6 to 9 o'clock

8.6 Postoperative Complications

Bleeding is about 1–2% and can occur immediately after the surgery; therefore sufficient hemostasis is essential during the surgery. Packing gauze for hemostasis, however, should be avoided as it obstructs the drainage. Urinary retention is a rare complication that can occur after spinal anesthesia like other anal surgeries, and it is mostly seen in men over age 50 and also in the cases with more than 1 L of fluid injected before and after the surgery. Intensive examination is essential if there is urinary retention with fever after normal urination, as it can be the signal for deteriorating of inflammation. In most cases, recurrence is from the fault of the surgical technique, and in the case of delayed treatment after the first symptom, recurrence is higher; therefore, anorectal abscess needs immediate treatment [27–29]. In the drainage process, through the incision wound, insert a finger, and check for any remaining abscess or hidden abscess in lattice form. There is high recurrence in horseshoe abscess as drainage wound is made in only one

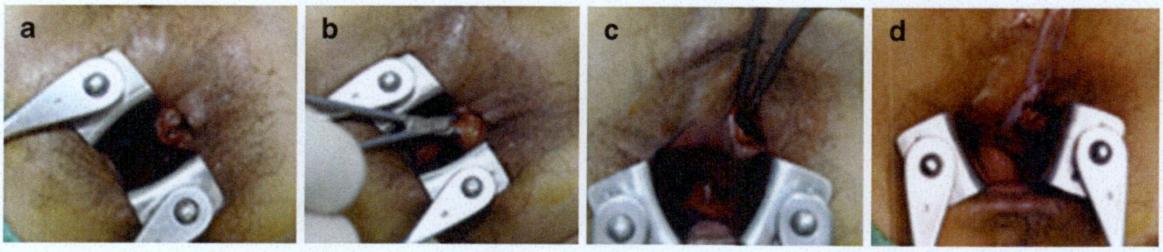

Fig. 8.5 Intersphincteric abscess with high extension. (**a**) Incision on the intersphincteric space. (**b**) Abscess drainage. (**c**) Confirmation of internal opening through the incision. (**d**) Seton application

side, and as time passes, inflammation occurs on the other side. It is difficult to consider abscess developing into anal fistula as a complication, because in most cases after drainage surgery in the perianal abscess, it develops into anal fistula and also in the cases with delayed treatment and complex abscess.

8.7 Anorectal Abscess in Special Cases

8.7.1 Perianal Abscess in Infant or Children

Perianal abscess in infant or children, in most cases, does not develop into anal fistula even with only simple incision and drainage, and it is known to heal easily [30]. But with recurrent abscess, cutting seton should be applied to avoid recurrence or developing into anal fistula together with the drainage.

8.7.2 Anorectal Infection in the Immunocompromised Patient

Anorectal abscess easily occurs in leukemia, lymphoma, and AIDS (acquired immune deficiency syndrome) patients and in about 5% of hospitalized patients [31]. It is closely related to blood neutrophil count, and the incidence is about 10% if it is less than 500/mm^3, but if it is higher, then it is lower than 1% [32]. In hospitalized patients with the above diseases and with suffering from discomfort in the perianal or perineum, intensive examination is needed as it can be a possibility of perianal abscess, with the avoidance of unnecessary digital examination or enema or mechanical device. If necessary, identify by MRI or CT and not ultrasonography. The severity of the original lesion is closely related to the prognosis; if the surgery is performed in the basis of general abscess, then the wound will not heal and can develop into sepsis by the spread of infection to the soft tissue, and therefore priority broad-spectrum antibiotic should be administered rather than surgical treatment. But if there is no response to antibiotic treatment or presence of definite fluctuation, you can carefully perform incision and drainage [33].

8.7.3 Necrotizing Anorectal Infection (Fournier's Gangrene)

This is a fatal disease accompanied with perineal pain, fever, chills, swelling, edema, and sudden inflammation within 2–5 days along the fascia [34]. It is most commonly seen in men around the age of 50, and the risk factors are DM, alcoholism, obesity, and immunocompromised patients. In the case with uncertain diagnosis, it is helpful to use CT to identify the primary lesion and the spread range of inflammation (Fig. 8.6) [35]. Immediate fluid treatment with broad-spectrum antibiotics and surgical excision of the devitalized tissue should be performed. Excision should be made over the necrotized tissue to the site where bleeding is identified and should not only be performed with a simple drainage. With the identified primary lesion, drain seton can be applied [36]. There is controversy on whether the fecal diversion helps the healing, but it should be made even for the protection of widely excised wound.

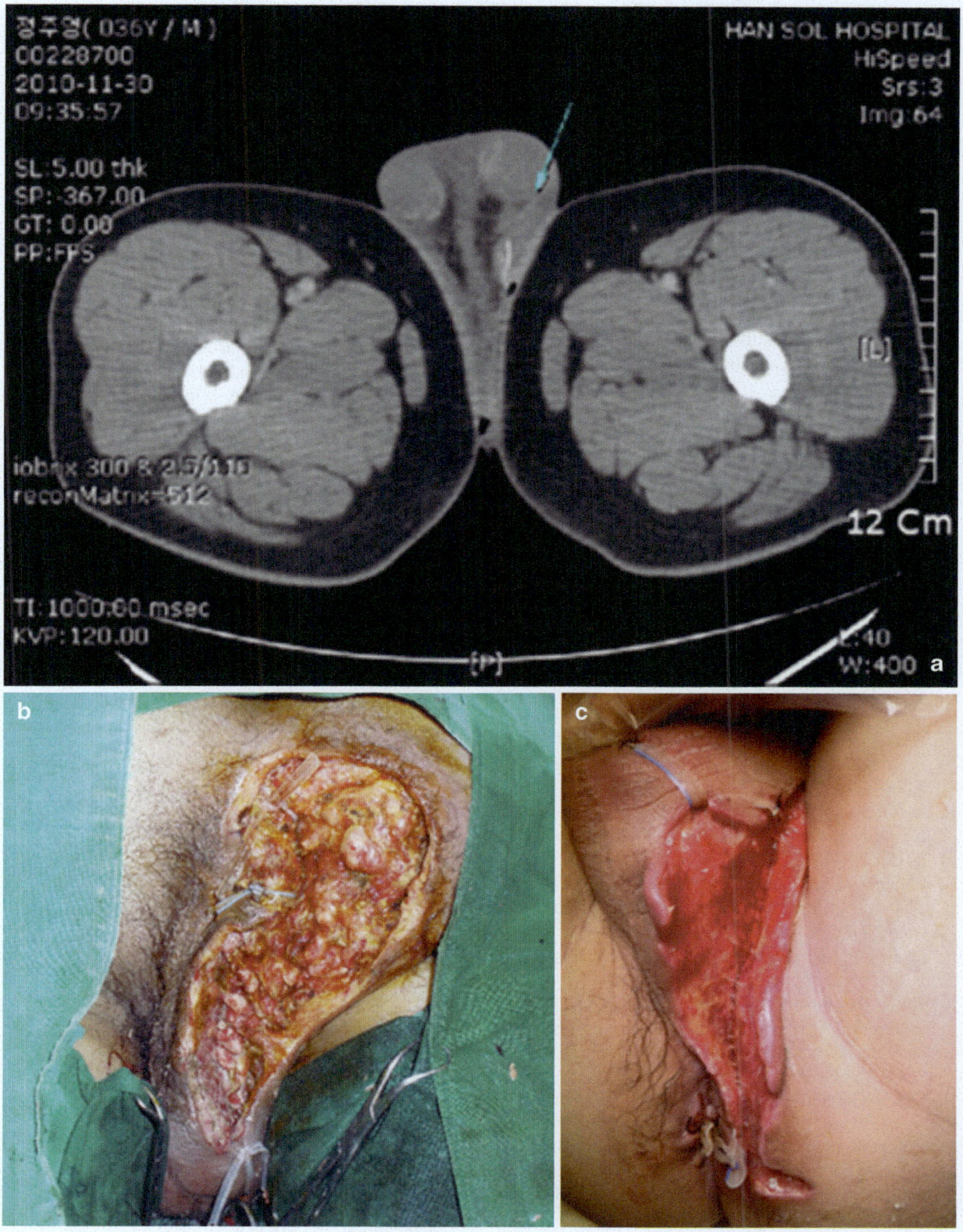

Fig. 8.6 Fournier's gangrene. (**a**) CT image of postoperative state; arrow points to 7 mm sized triangular low-attenuated lesion (abscess pocket) at the left scrotum. (**b**) Wide excision of scrotal lesion and seton application. (**c**) Postoperative follow-up state

References

1. Abcarian H. Anorectal infection: abscess-fistula. Clin Colon Rectal Surg. 2011;24:14–21.
2. Sneider EB, Maykel JA. Anal abscess and fistula. Gastroenterol Clin N Am. 2013;42:773–84.
3. Eisenhammer S. The internal anal sphincter and the anorectal abscess. Surg Gynecol Obstet. 1956;103:501–6.
4. Parks AG, Gordon PH, Hardcastle JD. A classification of fistula-in-ano. Br J Surg. 1976;63:1–12.
5. Schwartz DA, Loftus EV Jr, Tremaine WJ, Panaccione R, Harmsen WS, Zinsmeister AR, Sandborn WJ. The natural history of fistulizing Crohn's disease in Olmsted County, Minnesota. Gastroenterology. 2002;122:875–80.
6. Harper PH, Fazio VW, Lavery IC, Jagelman DG, Weakley FL, Farmer RG, Easley KA. The long-term outcome in Crohn's disease. Dis Colon Rectum. 1987;30:174–9.
7. Wiese DM, Schwartz DA. Managing Perianal Crohn's Disease. Curr Gastroenterol Rep. 2012;14:153–61.
8. Sordo-Mejia R, Gaertner WB. Multidisciplinary and evidence-based management of fistulizing perianal Crohn's disease. World J Gastrointest Pathophysiol. 2014;5:239–51.
9. Read DR, Abcarian H. A prospective survey of 474 patients with anorectal abscess. Dis Colon Rectum. 1979;22:566–8.
10. McElwain JW, MacLean MD, Alexander RM, Hoexter B. Guthrie Anorectal problems: experience with primary fistulectomy for anorectal abscess, a report of 1,000 cases. Dis Colon Rectum. 1975;18:646–9.
11. Visscher AP, Felt-Bersma RJ. Endoanal ultrasound in perianal fistulae and abscesses. Ultrasound Q. 2015;31:130–7.
12. Plaikner M, Loizides A, Peer S, Aigner F, Pecival D, Zbar A, Kremser C, Gruber H. Transperineal ultrasonography as a complementary diagnostic tool in identifying acute perianal sepsis. Tech Coloproctol. 2014;18:165–71.
13. Khati NJ, Sondel Lewis N, Frazier AA, Obias V, Zeman RK, Hill MC. CT of acute perianal abscesses and infected fistulae: a pictorial essay. Emerg Radiol. 2015;22:329–35.
14. Garcia-Granero A, Granero-Castro P, Frasson M, Flor-Lorente B, Carreño O, Espí A, Puchades I, Garcia-Granero E. Management of cryptoglandular supralevator abscesses in the magnetic resonance imaging era: a case series. Int J Color Dis. 2014;29:1557–64.
15. Steele SR, Kumar R, Feingold DL, Rafferty JL, Buie WD, Standards Practice Task Force of the American Society of Colon and Rectal Surgeons. Practice parameters for the management of perianal abscess and fistula-in-ano. Dis Colon Rectum. 2011;54:1465–74.
16. Sözener U, Gedik E, Kessaf Aslar A, Ergun H, Halil Elhan A, Memikoğlu O, Bulent Erkek A, Ayhan Kuzu M. Does adjuvant antibiotic treatment after drainage of anorectal abscess prevent development of anal fistulas? A randomized, placebo-controlled, double-blind, multicenter study. Dis Colon Rectum. 2011;54:923–9.
17. Tan KK, Koh DC, Tsang CB. Managing deep postanal space sepsis via an intersphincteric approach: our early experience. Ann Coloproctol. 2013;29:55–9.
18. Schouten WR, van Vroonhoven TJ. Treatment of anorectal abscess with or without primary fistulectomy. Results of a prospective randomized trial. Dis Colon Rectum. 1991;34:60–3.
19. Ho YH, Tan M, Chui CH, Leong A, Eu KW, Seow-Choen F. Randomized controlled trial of primary fistulotomy with drainage alone for perianal abscesses. Dis Colon Rectum. 1997;40:1435–8.
20. Quah HM, Tang CL, Eu KW, Chan SY, Samuel M. Meta-analysis of randomized clinical trials comparing drainage alone vs primary sphincter-cutting procedures for anorectal abscess-fistula. Int J Color Dis. 2006;21:602–9.
21. Oliver I, Lacueva FJ, Pérez Vicente F, Arroyo A, Ferrer R, Cansado P, Candela F, Calpena R. Randomized clinical trial comparing simple drainage of anorectal abscess with and without fistula track treatment. Int J Color Dis. 2003;18:107–10.
22. Malik AI, Nelson RL, Tou S. Incision and drainage of perianal abscess with or without treatment of anal fistula. Cochrane Database Syst Rev. 2010;(7):CD006827.
23. Hanley PH, Ray JE, Pennington EE, Grablowsky OM. Fistula-in-ano: a ten-year follow-up study of horseshoe-abscess fistula-in-ano. Dis Colon Rectum. 1976;19:507–15.
24. Browder LK, Sweet S, Kaiser AM. Modified Hanley procedure for management of complex horseshoe fistulae. Tech Coloproctol. 2009;13:301–6.
25. Ustynoski K, Rosen L, Stasik J, Riether R, Sheets J, Khubchandani IT. Horseshoe abscess fistula. Seton treatment. Dis Colon Rectum. 1990;33:602–5.
26. Rosen SA, Colquhoun P, Efron J, Vernava AM 3rd, Nogueras JJ, Wexner SD, Weiss EG. Horseshoe abscesses and fistulas: how are we doing? Surg Innov. 2006;13:17–21.
27. Hamadani A, Haigh PI, Liu IL, Abbas MA. Who is at risk for developing chronic anal fistula or recurrent anal sepsis after initial perianal abscess? Dis Colon Rectum. 2009;52:217–21.
28. Buchan R, Grace RH. Anorectal suppuration: the results of treatment and the factors influencing the recurrence rate. Br J Surg. 1973;60:537–40.
29. Vasilevsky CA, Gordon PH. The incidence of recurrent abscesses or fistula-in-ano following anorectal suppuration. Dis Colon Rectum. 1984;27:126–30.
30. Serour F, Somekh E, Gorenstein A. Perianal abscess and fistula-in-ano in infants: a different entity? Dis Colon Rectum. 2005;48:359–64.
31. Orkin BA, Smith LE. Perineal manifestations of HIV infection. Dis Colon Rectum. 1992;35:310–4.
32. Vanhueverzwyn R, Delannoy A, Michaux JL, Dive C. Anal lesions in hematologic diseases. Dis Colon Rectum. 1980;23:310–2.

33. Baker B, Al-Salman M, Daoud F. Management of acute perianal sepsis in neutropenic patients with hematological malignancy. Tech Coloproctol. 2014;18:327–33.
34. Laor E, Palmer LS, Tolia BM, Reid RE, Winter HI. Outcome prediction in patients with Fournier's gangrene. J Urol. 1995;154:89–92.
35. Anaya DA, Dellinger EP. Necrotizing soft-tissue infection: diagnosis and management. Clin Infect Dis. 2007;44:705–10.
36. Yang BL, Lin Q, Chen HJ, Gu YF, Zhu P, Sun XL, Shao WJ. Perianal necrotizing fasciitis treated with a loose-seton technique. Color Dis. 2012;14: e422–4.

9 Fistula-in-ano

Seung Han Kim

9.1 Introduction

Anal fistula is a chronic stage of anal inflammation with intermittent purulent discharge, in some cases with pain and edema. As 50% of anal abscesses do not heal spontaneously after incision and drainage, it develops into anal fistula; abscess can be divided into acute phase and anal fistula into chronic phase. Anal abscess is classified by the spaces between the tissues around the anorectum, and anal fistula is divided with the correlation between the fistula tract and the anal sphincter muscles. Prior to the treatment, surgeon should have accurate anatomical information between the fistula and anal sphincter to minimize the risk of postoperative incontinence. Also, to reduce the risk of incontinence, operative method is changing to minimize the sphincter damage compared to the past [1].

9.2 Pathophysiology

Ninety percent of anal fistula occurs with spontaneous rupture of anorectal abscess or after the incision and drainage. Abscess from other parts of the body can be cured from incision and drainage, but most of anorectal abscess develop into anal fistula. This is due to incomplete treatment of inflammatory focus started from the anal gland, and as the tract is formed from the fistula surrounded by the anorectal epithelial tissue, even with the incision and drainage, it is always in the condition of bacteria invasion through the tract [2]. There are much of fat tissues around the anorectum with low resistance to bacteria, and it is surrounded with muscular fibers running transversally and longitudinally, and as it is impossible to be stabilized due to the activity of the internal and external sphincter, longitudinal muscle, and levator muscle, it is easy for the inflammation to spread. The reason for anal fistula to occur mostly in the posterior side of the anus and in men is because the anal gland which is the origin of the inflammation is concentrated in the posterior side of the anus and there's more in men [3, 4]. However, in the case of perianal abscess that does not have connection with the anorectal wall, such as boil, hidradenitis suppurativa, and sebaceous adenitis, they are easily cured with incision and drainage. In anal fistula, anal crypt that is invaded by bacteria into the anal gland is referred to primary opening or internal opening, and where the abscess rupture is referred to secondary opening or external opening. Tuberculous fistula is often seen in tuberculosis patients. The incidence of tuberculous lesions detected by biopsy is about 5%. It is occurred in the anal canal infected by the tuberculosis of the swallowed sputum. Others are concurrent from Crohn's disease, ulcerative colitis, and rectal or anal cancer.

S. H. Kim (✉)
Colorectal Division, Department of Surgery,
Hansol Hospital, Seoul, South Korea

D. K. Lee (ed.), *Practices of Anorectal Surgery*, https://doi.org/10.1007/978-981-13-1447-6_9

9.3 Classification

To fully understand and treat anal fistula, it is necessary to understand the correlation between the fistula and surrounding anal sphincter and pelvic floor muscle (Fig. 9.1). In order to do this and to determine the treatment method, you have to have in your mind the planar description of fistula tract, which shows the primary opening, fistula passage and length, and the presence of the secondary opening and the dimensional description, which shows through which anorectal wall the fistula is reaching the perianal skin or mucosal surface. Park's classification is one of the most widely used in correlation with the fistula tract and the sphincter muscles, and this is classified by the relation between the fistula and the external sphincter muscle and generally classified into four categories depending on the presence of the secondary branch [5]. Some doctors from Japan and Korea follow Sumikoshi's classification [6], but we follow Park's classification.

9.3.1 Intersphincteric Fistula

Intersphincteric fistula is an inflammation spread to intersphincteric space without penetrating through the external sphincter, and Park classified it into six subtypes, but the highest incidence is from the opening in the direction of the perianal skin, and second highest is the high type which spread to the upper side; however, the incidence is not high. Intersphincteric fistula is about 30–40% of anal fistula.

9.3.2 Transsphincteric Fistula

Inflammation penetrating through the external sphincter, the fistula is located in the lower level of the puborectalis and is a typical form of ischiorectal abscess or deep postanal abscess developing into anal fistula. In very rare cases, blind tract may form on the upper portion of the levator muscles. This is generally caused by the careless iatrogenic penetration of the levator muscle during the drainage. Be cautious not to penetrate the levator muscle or the rectal wall with excessive strength in placing the probe as it can cause iatrogenic extrasphincteric fistula. As the fistula tract in transsphincteric type is generally formed at the right angle of the perianal skin from the primary opening and midline, a probe can be misplaced. To avoid this, probe from the primary opening or identify by dissecting along the fistula tract from the perianal secondary opening. There is simple form of transsphincteric fistula passing through the subcutaneous external sphincter. Transsphincteric fistula is about 40–50% of anal fistula.

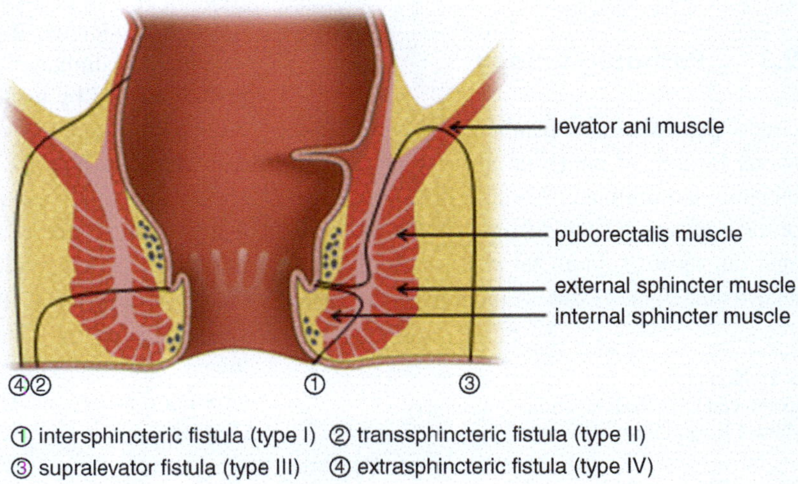

Fig. 9.1 Parks' classification of fistula-in-ano

9.3.3 Suprasphincteric Fistula

Ascending from intersphincteric space over the sphincter including puborectalis and, from there, penetrating the levator muscle and descend to ischiorectal and make opening in the perianal skin. Supralevator abscess should be drained to the rectum, but it can be iatrogenic fistula incorrectly drained to the perianal skin through ischiorectal fossa or in the case with abscess from supralevator space to the ischiorectal fossa descend spontaneously through the levator muscle, but the possibility is much high on the former. Suprasphincteric fistula is about 20% from Park's, but in general, it is within 2% of anal fistula [7].

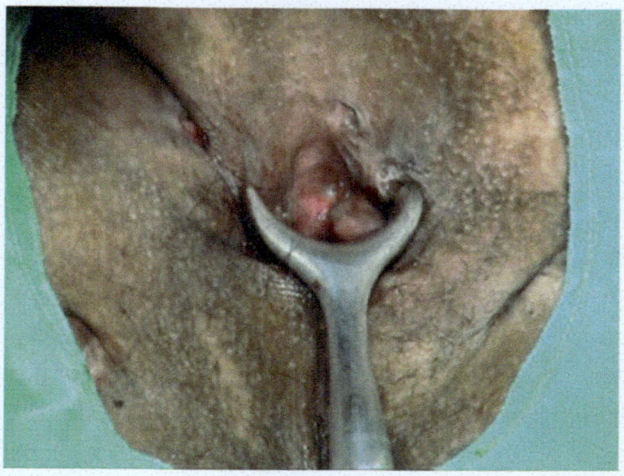

Fig. 9.2 Multiple secondary openings of horseshoe fistula. Internal opening at the 6 o'clock, and multiple secondary openings (2, 5, 10)

9.3.4 Extrasphincteric Fistula

This is the most rare case, with fistula formed in perianal skin through the levator muscle from the rectum, and it can develop from inflammatory bowel disease like Crohn's disease not like the inflammation origin from the anal gland or develop from pelvic inflammatory diseases and rectal wall injuries from fish bone.

Anal fistula also can be classified into simple or complex fistula. Simple fistula is a fistula with almost no risk of postoperative fecal incontinence, and complex is with risk of fecal incontinence. In general, complex fistula includes high-type transsphincteric fistula which includes over 30% of the external sphincter muscle, suprasphincteric fistula, extrasphincteric fistula, anterior side transsphincteric fistula in women, and fistula from after the malignant tumor surgery, Crohn's disease or accident, and fistula from the patients with fecal incontinence or chronic diarrhea [8, 9].

9.4 Diagnosis

Each patient describes their symptoms in various forms, but most of the patients have the experience in drainage treatment or have the memory of a burst of the abscess (Fig. 9.2). A feel of a lump or oozing, accompanying blood or they also say they have hemorrhoid. In most of the cases, anal fistula can be easily diagnosed by physical examination identifying the external opening. The most important for the doctors is to determine the correlation between the anal sphincter and where the internal opening is by examining the external opening. Based on the Goodall's rule, internal opening can be estimated from the 70% of the anal fistula. You can feel the fistula tract by digital examination and through anoscopy, rare, but you can sometimes identify the pus draining from the internal opening. If inflammatory bowel disease is suspected, it should be identified with proctoscopy. In some cases, internal opening or fistula tract is examined with imaging studies, but this is in the case of multiple external opening or recurrent fistula or uncertain internal opening from complex fistula by physical examination.

Fistulography was a typical evaluation study for the anal fistula in the past, but now it's no longer used, and CT fistulography is also an excellent method [10], but it is more complex compared to the MRI or ultrasonography and relatively inefficient due to the risk of radiation [11]. It is, however, helpful in extrasphincteric type, as you can identify the contrast medium coming out of the rectum [12]. Endoanal ultrasound can be easily used in outpatient clinic, and especially 3D US is very useful as it can be used during the operation and can identify the relation to anal sphincter in 3D. However, it is less useful in the cases with surgery history or scarring, stagnated undrained fluid, or history of anal injury. Also, it depends more on the ability of the clinician, and the negatives would be that, it is difficult to identify the deep fistula tract [13–15]. With MRI examination, it can be understood the anatomical structure of the anorectum without patient discomfort in the examination like ultrasonography or fistulography. It is useful in complex fistula which is difficult to examine with ultrasonography, or in the patients with severe scarring or have anatomical deformity from the previous operation. The advantage is that it can distinguish the postoperative recurrence from the scarring and inflammation from the previous operation. Also, this is an examination that can determine the presence of secondary tract and the evaluation of the fistula away from the anal canal and identify the primary opening most accurately [16–18].

9.5 Treatment

The target of the treatment is to prevent recurrence by removing the primary focus in the intersphincteric space and minimizing the sphincter damage and preserving its function to maintain anal function. It also involves making small wounds to promote quick healing. (Fig. 9.3). In most of the anal fistula, it needs surgical treatment, and in order to minimize the postoperative fecal incontinence or recurrence, there are diverse surgical methods introduced according to the cause and type of fistula, condition of the sphincter, and gender of the patient. In recurrent fistula, other treatment can be considered, but as it is very difficult to treat incontinence once occurred, it is more important to choose a surgical method that can minimize the sphincter damage than the recurrence [19, 20]. The cause of recurrence is in the cases with not knowing the relation between the fistula tract and the anal sphincter or not iden-

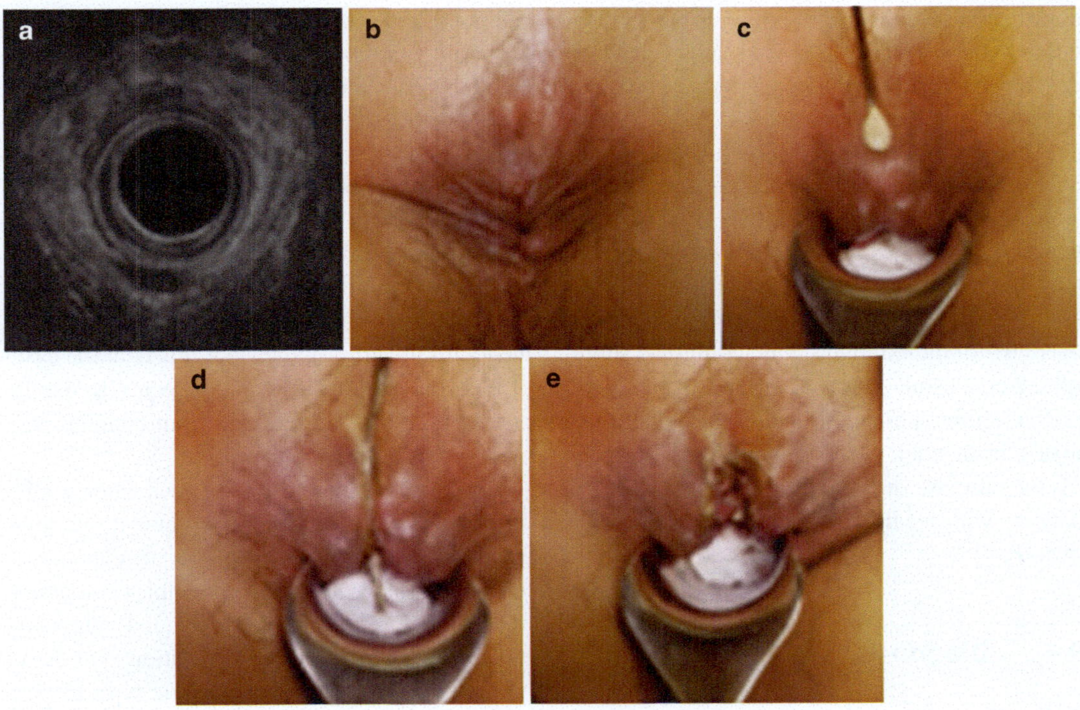

Fig. 9.3 Simple fistula in the direction of 6 o'clock. (**a**) Sonographic image of simple fistula. (**b**) Low-grade intersphincteric abscess at 6 o'clock. (**c**) Probing after incision and drainage. (**d**) Laying open. (**e**) After laying open

tified primary opening and without knowing the other special causes of the anal fistula [21]. Surgical method can be classified into sphincter division or sphincter saving. Anal fistulotomy or fistulectomy and cutting seton operation are in the former. Drain seton, advancement flap, fistula plug, and fibrin glue are in the sphincter-saving method. Sphincter division method can be performed in simple fistula, as the change of the anal function after the surgery is only minimal, but in the case of complex fistula, sphincter-saving method should be performed if possible. At first we will deal with simple fistula and complex fistula surgical methods.

9.5.1 Surgical Approach by the Complexity

In simple fistula, performing fistulotomy from external opening to internal opening has less damage to the sphincter and fast healing compared to the fistulectomy, and the recurrence rate is similar, about 5% [22, 23]. After the fistulotomy, by performing the marsupialization of the wound edge, it can help in fast healing and preserving the function of the anus. Even in simple fistula, seton application can be performed to reduce the risk of incontinence and keyhole deformity [24]. In the case of simple fistula with identified internal opening and accompanied by abscess, curative operation of fistula and drainage should be planned with immediate incision. Lay opening is referring to incise and open. The means of laying open procedure for fistula are to leave it as the tract is opened, complete curettage on epithelialized fistula tract without fistulectomy method, complete curettage and fistulectomy on hard fistula, and complete fistulectomy of fistula tract [22]. Causes of delay in the healing after fistulotomy can be the remaining epithelialized anal gland, scar tissue, and flaccid granulation tissue; therefore, it is recommended to choose appropriate method depending on the cases to remove the causes.

Anatomical structure of complex fistula can be identified in most cases with using the probe in the operation room, but using ultrasonography or MRI to identify the relation between the external sphincters prior to the surgery can be a great help in setting surgical plan. Based on Park's theory, anal gland starts from internal opening and penetrates internal sphincter and ends in the intersphincteric space. Outside tract from the external sphincter is the secondary outcome of the anal gland infection (Fig. 9.4). From there, excise several mm of internal sphincter together with the mucosa from internal opening and extract anal gland followed by partial internal sphincterectomy, and it is considered to be naturally healed even with the fistula in the outer side of the external sphincter. If concerned about draining the remained fistula, then it can be done by coring out from the external opening. According to Parks, the recurrence rate of this procedure is 9% which is fairly high. It is called as sphincter-saving procedure, an improved transformed surgical method; one method is excising primary opening and removing fistula tract from the secondary opening then suture the wound in the anal canal by advancement flap, and the other method is excising primary opening and coring out fistula from the secondary opening then suture the wound in the anal canal. After the

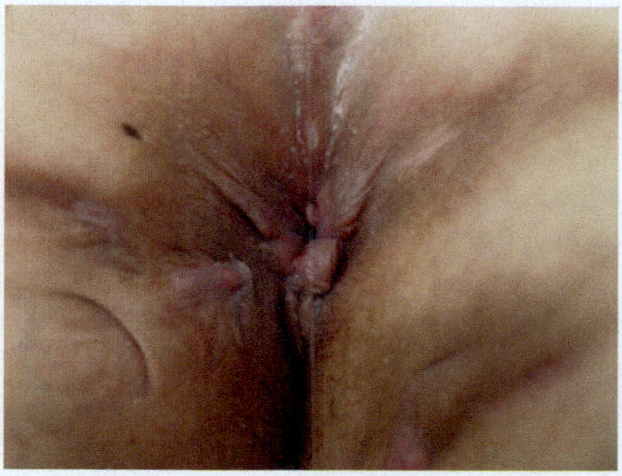

Fig. 9.4 Multiple external opening (2′, 3′) in the complex fistula

complete excision on the fistula penetrating primary opening and internal sphincter, suture internal sphincter with chromic catgut. Suture is mainly for the hemostasis. In some cases, success rate is high with decompression of the increased pressure of the anal canal, which is incising posterior side of the anus. Seton application is most widely used in complex fistula; seton is applied along the fistula tract, and fibrosis occurs around the fistula due to the foreign body reaction and even with the incision of the remaining muscle or muscle incision by the seton application, as it has limited muscular damage and the risk of fecal incontinence is limited [25–28]. Seton is also used as a mark in a staged transection to identify the degree of the muscle to be cut. Recurrence rate is low, but the risk of fecal incontinence is higher than sphincter-saving procedure [29, 30]. Generally in the case of high-type transsphincteric fistula or complex fistula, staged fistulotomy is performed by cutting seton. In some cases, even with low-type transsphincteric fistula, if there is pre- and postoperative poor sphincter function, seton application is used without immediate fistulotomy. In cutting seton, in some cases, it drops out naturally, but in most cases, staged fistulotomy is performed between 4 and 6 weeks. And sometimes prior to the fistulotomy, in the case of too much remaining the external sphincter, seton is tightened or drain seton is applied and fistulotomy is performed later or the seton is removed only, the functional damage is much less [31]. In some cases, to expect better functional outcome from reducing the external sphincter damage, fistulectomy to intersphincteric and from intersphincteric, apply cutting seton in the inner side, and drain seton in the outer side. However, in any cases, the seton application in complex fistula is not an actual means of sphincter-saving procedure, but it's just to reduce the sphincter damage.

9.5.2 Surgical Approach by Park's Classification

9.5.2.1 Intersphincteric Fistula

Based on the simple fistula treatment, laying open all fistula tract with identifying the location of the internal opening and the passage of the fistula (Fig. 9.5). In high-type intersphincteric fistula, incise the internal sphincter to the rectal wall of the highest point of the fistula tract, and if there is inflammation, it is recommended to apply seton and incise afterward. Be cautious with the hemostasis on the incision site. Fistulotomy is considered to be functionally better than the fistulectomy, but if the cause of anal fistula is suspected to be from other disease, then biopsy should be performed with fistulectomy.

9.5.2.2 Transsphincteric Fistula

Most of the transsphincteric fistula is low type; therefore, there is no anal dysfunction after fistulotomy, and in the case of high-type transsphincteric fistula, the main sphincter function is known to be maintained if the puborectalis muscle is preserved. But 1/3 of the patients had minor bowel control disorder and fecal soiling symptom [31]. Especially in the case of elderly or women patients with anterior anal fistula, fistulotomy can cause severe dysfunction of the anus. In the case of fistulotomy, if the included range of the external sphincter is over 30% seton application or other

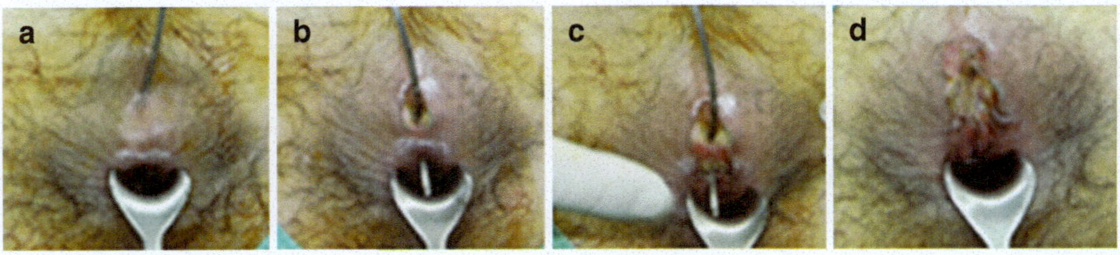

Fig. 9.5 Fistulotomy for intersphincteric fistula. (**a**) Probing through the external opening. (**b**) Confirmation of the internal opening at 6 o'clock. (**c**) Laying open of the fistula tract. (**d**) Unroofing state

sphincter-saving method should be chosen, due to the high risk of postoperative fecal incontinence. However, these surgical methods have the advantage of minimizing sphincter damage, but the negative side is that, still, recurrence rate is relatively high. Seton can be applied with tying the muscle included in the fistula tract and during the 4 weeks' time with fibrosis around the sphincter, maintaining sphincter function can be expected, but it is not a complete sphincter-saving surgery, and there is various degree of postoperative sphincter damage. If there is no inflammation due to stabilized fistula, fistulectomy can be performed, and immediate sphincter closing suture can be performed (Fig. 9.6).

9.5.2.3 Suprasphincteric Fistula

This form of fistula not only includes puborectalis but also includes the complete external sphincter; therefore, if all of the fistula tracts are incised, fecal incontinence cannot be avoided. Therefore, treatment should be chosen within the several sphincter-saving methods. In general, to remove primary lesion, it is advisable to incise internal sphincter of the lower part of the primary opening and make sufficient drain wound and apply seton on the remaining external sphincter. Other methods like fistula incision and simple suture or muscle-filling method or mucosa advancement flap can be considered, but the recurrence rate is high. In suprasphincteric fistula method, it should be performed through sufficient pre- and intraoperative evaluation and after determining the accurate relation with the sphincter muscle. In some cases, it is mistaken with transsphincteric fistula; therefore, unnecessary seton application in the levator muscle should be avoided.

9.5.2.4 Extrasphincteric Fistula

Extrasphincteric fistula is mainly caused by iatrogenic cause and can occur from complication of rectal injury or pelvic sepsis or inflammatory bowel disease (Fig. 9.7). Most of the extrasphincteric fistula other than Crohn's disease is treated with excision of the primary opening and advancement flap method, but recurrence rate is higher compared to the other types of fistula. Prior to the surgery, intestinal lavage and antibiotic injection are needed, and after the surgery, 2 days of NPO and 3 days of bowel restrain are needed.

9.5.2.5 Horseshoe Fistula

In horseshoe fistula, inflammation spreads in cylindrical and tends to have another secondary opening on the left and right side and sometimes on only one side. It can be seen in intersphincteric, transsphincteric, or suprasphincteric fistula, and transsphincteric fistula originated from the posterior side of the anus is most common. Internal opening is generally located in posterior midline of the anal canal and stretches out to the ischioanal fossa of both sides and form U-shaped fistula (Fig. 9.8). It is rare but there are cases having internal opening in the anterior. Traditional treatment method is to incise all anal fistula and internal opening, but then it needs longer time for wound healing and it can lead to anal deformity or functional disorder. For more saving methods, there is modified Hanley method, incising posterior internal sphincter and excising primary focus

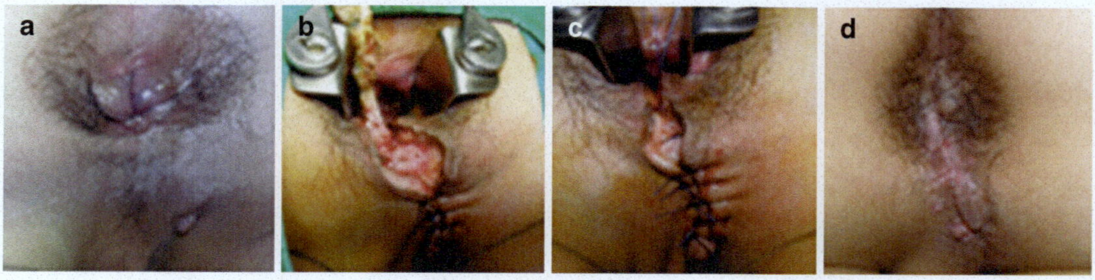

Fig. 9.6 Transsphincteric fistula. (**a**) High-type transsphincteric fistula with external opening in the 11 o'clock. (**b**) Coring out of fistula tract. (**c**) After coring out and seton application, partial external wide wound is sutured partially for wound healing. (**d**) Healing state after operation

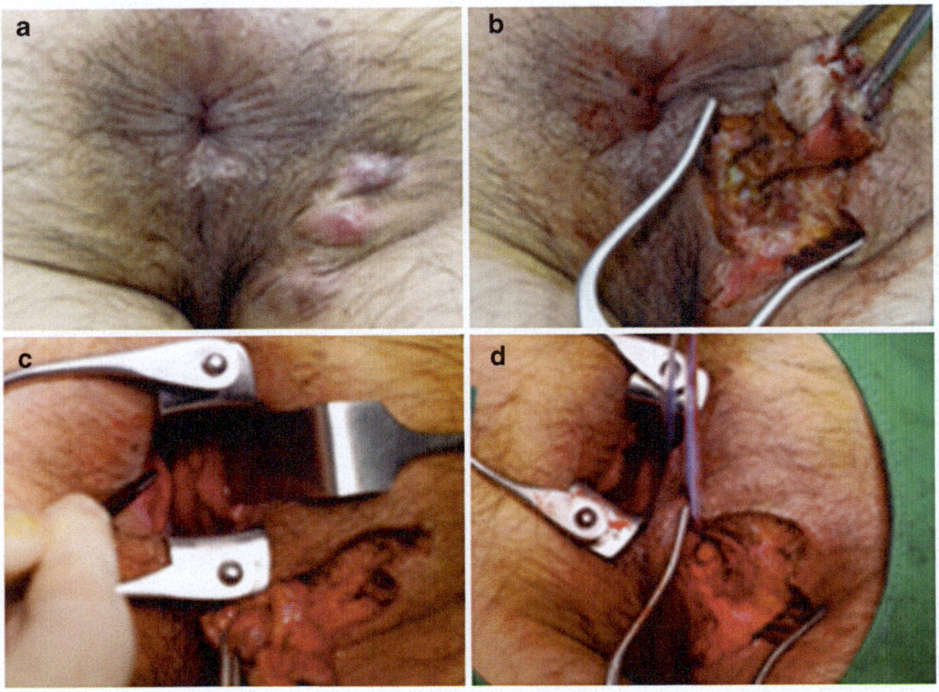

Fig. 9.7 Extrasphincteric fistula. (**a**) Extrasphincteric fistula with external opening in 10 o'clock. (**b**, **c**) Coring out the fistula tract, including external opening. (**d**) Seton application to the remaining external sphincters

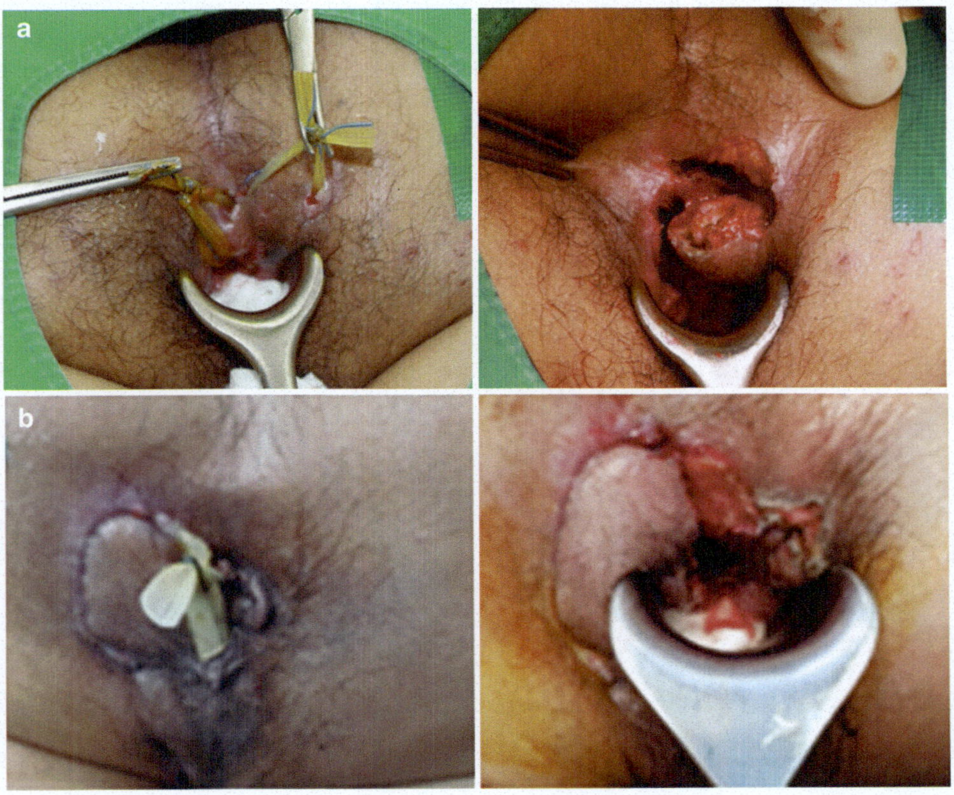

Fig. 9.8 Horseshoe fistula. (**a**) Postoperative state – seton. Horseshoe fistula with external opening on left side. The internal opening at 6 o'clock and the external opening at 9 o'clock are seton applied, respectively. (**b**) Unroofing of all remained fistula tracts after seton removal

of the intersphincteric space and deep postanal space and curettage by widening external opening and then the drainage (Fig. 9.9) [32, 33]. From this, better anal function can be expected by reducing the external sphincter damage.

9.5.3 Treatment of the Internal Opening (Primary Opening)

9.5.3.1 Identifying Internal Opening

Ninety percent of the low-type intersphincteric fistula have external opening in the posterior side of the anus, and about 60% here have easy identification of internal opening. In order to identify internal opening, first, insert finger into the rectum and check for hardness or tenderness on pressure, and place crypt hook in the suspicious anal crypt and identify whether there is connection with external opening. Infected anal crypt is larger and located in posterior midline. With pressure, pus can be drained from the affected anal crypt, and also it can accompany whitish scar or hypertrophic papilla. In the case with difficulty in identifying internal opening, insert slim silicon tube and inject 10 cc of saline solution lightly mixed with methylene blue (Fig. 9.10). Also, with the injection of saline solution in the mucosa of the suspicious anal crypt area, affected crypt will sink.

9.5.3.2 Treatment for Unidentified Internal Opening

In the case with difficulty in identifying internal opening even with many methods, and also in the case with suspicion to the primary lesion, complete fistulotomy cannot be performed. In this case, excise including the two to three suspicious anal crypt and lay open or incise wide in the external opening and follow-up with examination.

9.5.3.3 High Internal Opening

In case of internal opening being higher than the dentate line and non-clear relation with the puborectalis muscle, incision and laying open will leave anxiety in puborectalis saving. It is recommanded to apply seton and tie internal and external opening loosely with rubber band or silk thread, and, later, pull this thread and tighten the sphincter and incision, and to lay open by checking the relation between the internal opening and anorectal ring [21].

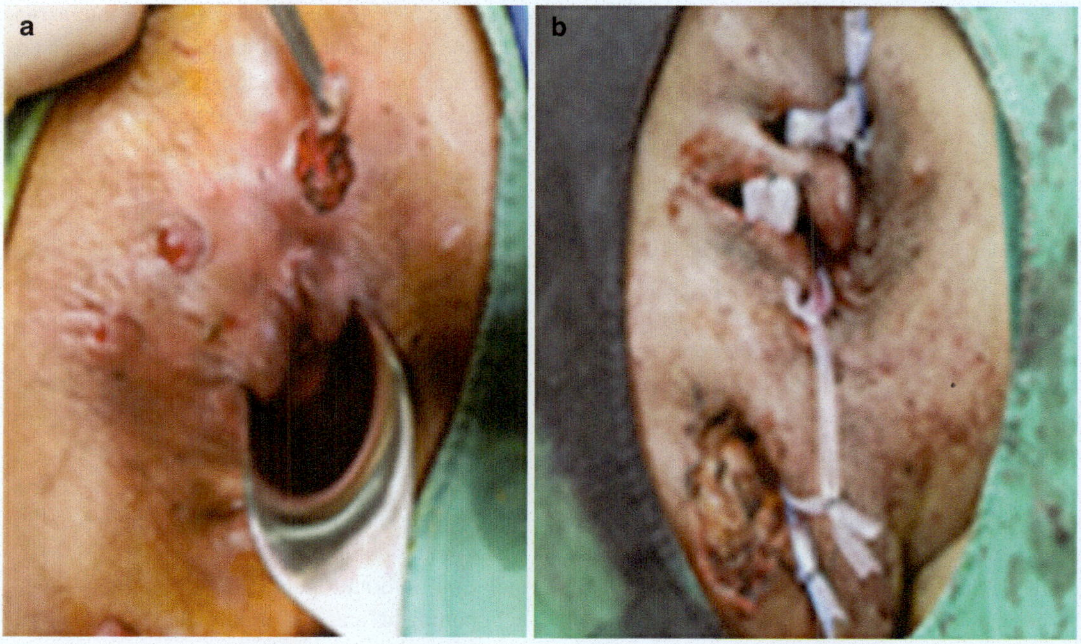

Fig. 9.9 Complex fistula. (**a**) Multiple transsphincteric fistulas at 1 o'clock, 5 o'clock, and 6 o'clock. (**b**) Seton application after coring out each fistulas

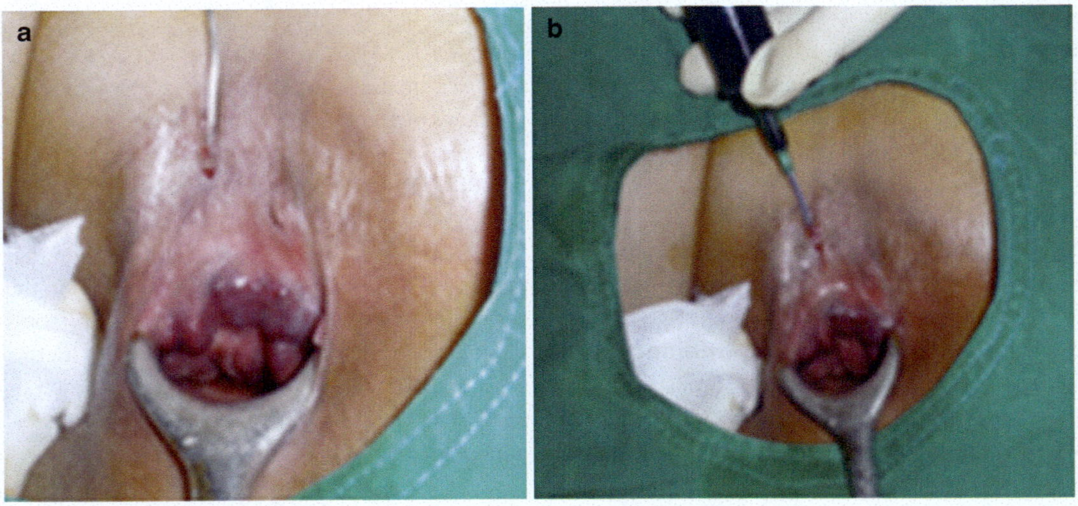

Fig. 9.10 Identifying internal opening. (**a**) Probing through the external opening. (**b**) Injection of saline solution with methylene blue

9.5.4 Sphincter-Preserving Operation

9.5.4.1 Advancement Flap

There are two methods in advancement flap, using the rectum and perianal skin. Endorectal advancement flap showed good outcome from rectovaginal fistula treatment; therefore, it is applied to anal fistula [34–36]. Flap is made in U shape from the anal canal to the 4–5 cm of lower rectum including the internal opening. Excise a part of the flap that has internal opening. Next steps are coring out or curettage of fistula and then suture internal sphincter of the internal opening. Interrupted suture is performed in the anal incision site and the edge by pulling the flap using 3.0 Vicryl. Advantage of this surgery is that there is no incision in sphincter and no wound in perianal area and less pain and to avoid the anal deformity and fast wound healing. But there is controversy on the thickness of the rectal flap (whether to include the muscle or make flap in the submucosal layer), whether to make temporary enterostomy, whether to use drain, up to where the flap should be pulled down and sutured. The factors that can affect the treatment evaluation are surgery history and method, cause of fistula, use of steroid prior to the surgery, postoperative use of anti-diarrheal agent, antibiotics, fecal diversion enterostomy, patient gender, age, and BMI, but in general, it is known to not affect the outcome. The disadvantages of this procedure are that the patients can suffer from rectal mucosal ectropion and seepage due to the descent of rectal mucosa to the distal anal canal. In cutaneous advancement flap, anal crypt around internal opening including the anal mucosa and fistula is incised, and then the defected area of the internal sphincter is sutured [37–40]. You can make V-Y form or house form of cutaneous flap, and pull into the anal canal and suture in the rectal mucosa to cover the location of the previous internal opening. It is better to make a wide drain wound for external opening drainage. The base of the flap is made twice wider than the apex. In general, an appropriate base of flap is about 1.5 cm and the length 3 cm, but it can be made bigger according to the circumstances. Surgical technique is easier than the advancement flap in the rectal mucosa, but it is reported to have higher recurrence rate. Another method is making distal flap by incising lower rectal mucosa of the upper dentate line. The shape of the flap is inverted or U shaped, and it is composed of mucosa, submucosal layer, and part of internal sphincter. When flap is ready and complete, you can excise distal flap including internal opening, and then ligate internal opening area and suture the flap with the incision area of lower rectum and cover the internal opening completely. In some cases, there can be tension in the anal gland skin. In such a case, it is necessary to relieve the tension by incising subcutaneous layer.

9.5.4.2 Ligation of Intersphincteric Fistula (LIFT)

For this surgery, it is very important to have fistula in stabilized condition after the fibrosis, and it is appropriate for high-type transsphincteric fistula [41]. Surgical technique: it should be performed in prone jackknife position under spinal anesthesia, and you must identify external opening, and incise the intersphincteric space about 3 cm in length and approach fistula. It is good to use an lone star retractor to secure the vision and dissect avoiding damage to fistula. Using bent forceps, you can ligate with 2–0 Vicryl pulling fistula and attaching it closely to the internal and external sphincter, and cut the center (Fig. 9.11). Curettage outer side of fistula and widen the area of external opening is needed for better drainage. After surgery the patient should be given antibiotics and bulking agent. Modified surgical techniques are sometimes used, incising internal sphincter along the fistula from internal opening, but traditional surgical technique is necessary for preserving the sphincter [42]. The success rate reported from the meta-analysis is about 70%, and the failure factors reported are obesity, smoking, recurrent anal fistula, and long fistula [43, 44]. In the case of failure in this surgical method, the cause could be the insufficient drainage and inflammation in the sphincter from ultrasonography, and it can be treated with simple incision [45, 46].

9.5.4.3 Fibrin Glue

From the early 1990, fibrin sealant started to be used, as there's advantage of convenient usage, repeated usage, and there is no sphincter damage [47, 48]. But due to high recurrence rate compared to the early stage, it is now rarely used in Korea. In general, fibrin sealant is composed of two materials: fibrinogen concentrates and thrombin. To stabilize fibrin monomer, Factor XIII is added, and to prevent fibrinolysis, aprotinin is added. It is known to promote healing by injecting fibrin sealant into fistula to form collagen [47]. In surgical technique, it is performed in prone jackknife position under spinal anesthesia; you can curette fistula tract after the definite identification of internal opening. You should stop the surgery in the case of remained abscess or secondary branch, and apply seton. After injecting the needle carefully into the internal opening until it is seen through the external opening, then, you can slowly pull back and inject fibrin glue to the external opening. After 1 minute, the glue is hardened and stabilized. There is no need for antibiotics after the surgery, but excessive activ-

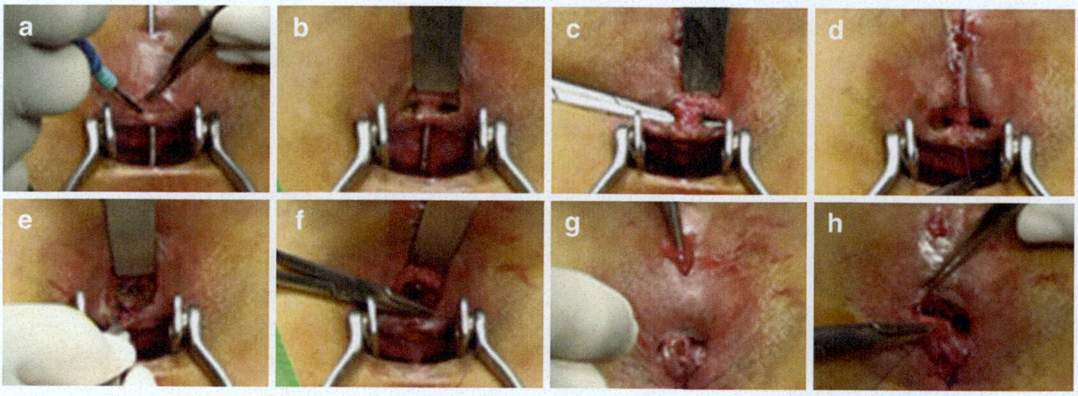

Fig. 9.11 Ligation of intersphincteric fistula (LIFT). (**a** and **g**) Through the external opening, probing to the internal opening to identify the correct fistula tract. (**b**) After incision in about 3 cm along the intersphincteric groove, dissection through the intersphincteric space to the tract. (**c**) Identify the fistula tract while avoiding damage to internal and external sphincters. (**d** and **e**) Ligation of fistula tract in the intersphincteric space. (**h**) Suture of intersphincteric incision site

ity or sitz bath should be avoided [49]. It is not certain but the failure factors can be the type of fibrin sealant used, incomplete removal of granulation tissue, insufficient fill up of fistula tract with fibrin sealant, and the length of fistula, and the success rate is lower in complex fistula [47]. The success rate reported from meta-analysis is about 50%, and it is not an appropriate primary treatment for complex fistula as it is difficult to probe to the internal opening along the fistula tract [50, 51]. Considering the expense and success rate, it is difficult to be used in Korea under the DRG system, but in some cases, Permacol (Tissue Science Lab) injection is used in Korea.

9.5.4.4 Fistula Plug

In 2006, Johnson and others reported 87% success rate in the attempt of filling the fistula with biological materials (Surgisis® Cook Surgical) on 15 patients. Then Surgisis anal fistula plug (AFP, Cook Surgical) was introduced, and it acts as tissue scaffold promoting the healing of fistula by stimulating the host fibroblast. Surgical technique is performed in prone jackknife position under spinal anesthesia; you can curette fistula tract with definite identification of internal opening through the external opening. You should stop the surgery in the case of remained abscess or secondary branch, and apply seton. In the next step you can dip the plug in the physiological saline about 3–5 minutes and then tie distal part with thread and pull out internal opening through the external opening and cut the remaining fistula. The internal opening area is sutered with 2–0 Vicryl and closed, and slightly widen the external opening area for better drainage. The overall success rate is lower than 50%, and the success rate is higher with longer fistula [52, 53], but under the circumstances, like fibrin glue, it is difficult to be used in Korea.

9.6 Fistula in Special Cases

9.6.1 Fistula in Infant

Infant anal fistula has high incidence for first occurrence in patients less than 3 months after birth. Most of the cases are low type, and the incidence of occurring in the lateral is higher than adult. In girls, it is more seen in anterior or posterior than the lateral. It occurred more in the baby fed with milk than the breastfed, and the natural healing is relatively high.

The cause of infant anal fistula is the infection in the anal crypt and anal gland, and this spreads into the surrounding subcutaneous tissue and forms abscess which develops to anal fistula with natural rupture or incision and drainage. The reason for infant anal fistula occurring mostly in the lateral is because of the incomplete anal sphincter, the infection usually occurs in the lateral side as anodermal transitional zone is susceptible to the pressure with feces instead of the sphincter, and the less rectal reflexion compared to the adults, prominent protrusion of the Morgagni gland in infants, frequent water stool, development abnormalities in the anal crypt and anal gland, and low production of lgA can be the reasons. Gastrointestinal immunization is completed about 1 year after birth, but the incidence of anal fistula can be high if the infant is milk fed rather than breast fed, as it can make the protective mechanism in gastrointestinal immunization lower. However, as the gastrointestinal immunization is completed 1 year after birth, after 1 year it can be naturally healed, and the occurrence of anal fistula is rare in the age after 1 year [54–57].

Yazbeck et al. reported that although 92% of fistulas in infants are preceded by a perianal abscess, only 42% of perianal abscess will result in fistula formation. Infantile fistula treated by either fistulotomy or fistulectomy can be expected good result [58].

9.6.2 Crohn's Disease Fistula

In Crohn's disease, anal fistula is different from the general anal fistula originating from the anal gland; inflammation passes through the rectal wall and develops into abscess. The occurrence is higher in the large intestine invaded by Crohn's disease than small intestine, and the treatment differs to the complexity of anal fistula and the degree of rectal inflammation from Crohn's disease. Also, in the patients with already diagnosed

Crohn's disease, multidisciplinary approach is necessary prior to the curative treatment. In the case of fistula with different forms other than the general shape, the possibility of accompanying Crohn's disease should then be considered. In the case of abscess, it is better to perform incision and drainage preferentially, then apply drain seton. Even with simple anal fistula, with Crohn's disease, fistulotomy or fistulectomy [59–61] should not be performed. In anal fistula, if drain seton is applied and maintained for long time, fistula can naturally close with active medical treatment like infliximab; therefore, it is advisable to remove only the seton as the inflammation subsides and to continue the medical treatment [62]. Recently, for the treatment of complex fistula, stem cell separated from the fat cell is cultured and used for the treatment, but it should be observed with time whether it can be a help to Crohn's disease fistula [63, 64].

9.7 Postoperative Complications

In most cases, there is no need to restrict patient's dietary, but warm sitz bath should be performed from the next day after the operation. However, in the case of patients with sphincter-saving method, bowel movement is restrained for 2–3 days after the operation, and warm sitz bath is performed after the first defecation. Initially, patients should be examined every week through outpatient clinic to check operation wound, then, to check the recovery process. Postoperative recovery period varies from 4 weeks to months depending on the degree of complexity of the anal fistula.

9.7.1 Anal Deformity and Displacement

If all of the anal fistula tract is opened while moving forward to anterior or lateral side of the anus, the deeper the penetration of the sphincter area, it can lead to severe anal deformity and displacement. But if the fistula is in the direction of posterior side, no severe deformity or displacement will occur even fully opened. It can be left open if there is no anal dysfunction even with the anal deformity and displacement; however, if cosmetic improvement is needed, anoplasty should be performed. Major cause of anal deformity and displacement is sphincter cut, and especially in horse shape fistula, with complete incision along the fistula, deformity cannot be avoided.

9.7.2 Fecal Incontinence

Even with 2–3 cuts at once in the subcutaneous layer from the external anal sphincter, it does not cause great disorder. However, when superficial and deep external sphincter muscles are cut from anterior or lateral side of the anus, it causes fecal incontinence due to the weakening of anal contraction. It is known to not cause severe fecal incontinence unless the puborectalis is cut in the posterior midline. But as the anal canal function differs in patients, it is inappropriate to generalize. Especially it should be cautious with old-aged or women patients, as the anterior anus is vulnerable. Therefore, prior to the operation, there should be an adequate evaluation through anal function test including the anal manometry.

9.7.3 Recurrence

Recurrence occurs with the failure in identifying the primary opening or with not recognizing the dilated secondary fistula to the lateral or upper side. The recurrence rate is 4–40%, and it differs depending on the surgical method. Also, recurrence occurs with a special cause like tuberculosis or Crohn's disease.

9.8 Summary

The most important in anal fistula surgery is to identify the primary focus and to remove the primary focus of the intersphincteric inflammation. For the large and deep anal fistula, sufficient drain wound is essential.

References

1. Blumetti J, Abcarian A, Quinteros F, Chaudhry V, Prasad L, Abcarian H. Evolution of treatment of fistula in ano. World J Surg. 2012;36:1162–7.
2. Parks A. Pathogenesis and treatment of fistula-in-ano. Br Med J. 1961;1:463–9.
3. Eglitis J. The gland of the anal canal in man. Ohio J Sci. 1961;61:65–79.
4. Seow-Choen F, Ho JM. Histoanatomy of anal glands. Dis Colon Rectum. 1994;37:1215–8.
5. Parks A, Gordon P, Hardcastle J. A classification of fistula-in-ano. BJS. 1976;63:1–12.
6. Sumikoshi Y, Takano M, Okada M, Kiratuka J, Sato S. New classification of fistulas and its application to the operations. Am J Proctol. 1974;25(3):72.
7. Sileri P, Cadeddu F, D'Ugo S, Franceschilli L, Del Vecchio Blanco G, De Luca E, Calabrese E, Capperucci SM, Fiaschetti V, Milito G, Gaspari AL. Surgery for fistula-in-ano in a specialist colorectal unit: a critical appraisal. BMC Gastroenterol. 2011;11:120–6.
8. Fazio VW. Complex anal fistulae. Gastroenterol Clin N Am. 1987;16:93–114.
9. Sangwan YP, Rosen L, Riether RD, Stasik JJ, Sheets JA, Khubchandani IT. Is simple fistula-in-ano simple? Dis Colon Rectum. 1994;37:885–9.
10. Liang C, Jiang W, Zhao B, Zhang Y, Du Y, Lu Y. CT imaging with fistulography for perianal fistula: does it really help the surgeon? Clin Imaging. 2013;37:1069–76.
11. Pomerri F, Dodi G, Pintacuda G, Amadio L, Muzzio PC. Anal endosonography and fistulography for fistula-in-ano. Radiol Med. 2010;115:771–83.
12. Weisman RI, Orsay CP, Pearl RK, Abcarian H. The role of fistulography in fistula-in-ano. Report of five cases. Dis Colon Rectum. 1991;34:181–4.
13. Choen S, Burnett S, Bartram CI, Nicholls RJ. Comparison between anal endosonography and digital examination in the evaluation of anal fistulae. Br J Surg. 1991;78:445–7.
14. Subasinghe D, Samarasekera DN. Comparison of preoperative endoanal ultrasonography with intraoperative findings for fistula in ano. World J Surg. 2010;34:1123–7.
15. Toyonaga T, Tanaka Y, Song JF, Katori R, Sogawa N, Kanyama H, Hatakeyama T, Matsushima M, Suzuki S, Mibu R, Tanaka M. Comparison of accuracy of physical examination and endoanal ultrasonography for preoperative assessment in patients with acute and chronic anal fistula. Tech Coloproctol. 2008;12:217–23.
16. Lunniss PJ, Barker PG, Sultan AH, Armstrong P, Reznek RH, Bartram CI, Cottam KS, Phillips RK. Magnetic resonance imaging of fistula-in-ano. Dis Colon Rectum. 1994;37:708–18.
17. Lunniss PJ, Armstrong P, Barker PG, Reznek RH, Phillips RK. Magnetic resonance imaging of anal fistulae. Lancet. 1992;340(8816):394–6.
18. Buchanan G, Halligan S, Williams A, Cohen CR, Tarroni D, Phillips RK, Bartram CI. Effect of MRI on clinical outcome of recurrent fistula-in-ano. Lancet. 2002;360(9346):1661–2.
19. Mazier WP. The treatment and care of anal fistulas: a study of 1,000 patients. Dis Colon Rectum. 1971;14:134–44.
20. Garcia-Aguilar J, Belmonte C, Wong WD, Goldberg SM, Madoff RD. Anal fistula surgery. Dis Colon Rectum. 1996;39:723–9.
21. Thompson H. Wound healing and fistula-in-ano. Lond Clin Med J. 1966;7:55.
22. Abcarian H. The 'lay open'technique. Anal fistula: surgical evaluation and management. London: Chapman & Hall Medical; 1996. p. 73–80.
23. Kronborg O. To lay open or excise a fistula-in-ano: a randomized trial. Br J Surg. 1985;72(12):970.
24. Takano M, Fujuyoshi T, Hidaka H, Naito H. Sphincter-preserving operation for low intersphincteric fistula. Nippon Daicho Komonbyo Gakkai Zasshi. 1986;39(1):1–9.
25. Van Tets W, Kuijpers J. Seton treatment of perianal fistula with high anal or rectal opening. Br J Surg. 1995;82(7):895–7.
26. Pearl RK, Andrews JR, Orsay CP, Weisman RI, Prasad ML, Nelson RL, et al. Role of the seton in the management of anorectal fistulas. Dis Colon Rectum. 1993;36(6):573–9.
27. Graf W, Påhlman L, Ejerblad S. Functional results after seton treatment of high transsphincteric anal fistulas. Eur J Surg Acta chirurgica. 1995;161(4):289–91.
28. Kuypers HC. Use of the seton in the treatment of extrasphincteric anal fistula. Dis Colon Rectum. 1984;27(2):109–10.
29. Isbister WH, Al Sanea N. The cutting seton. Dis Colon Rectum. 2001;44(5):722–7.
30. Limura E, Giordano P. Modern management of anal fistula. World J Gastroenterol. 2015;21:12.
31. Thomson JP, Ross AH. Can the external anal sphincter be preserved in the treatment of trans-sphincteric fistula-in-ano? Int J Color Dis. 1989;4:247–50.
32. Hanley PH. Conservative surgical correction of horseshoe abscess and fistula. Dis Colon Rectum. 1965;8(5):364–8.
33. Ustynoski K, Rosen L, Stasik J, Riether R, Sheets J, Khubchandani IT. Horseshoe abscess fistula. Dis Colon Rectum. 1990;33(7):602–5.
34. Hyman N. Endoanal advancement flap repair for complex anorectal fistulas. Am J Surg. 1999;178(4):337–40.
35. Joo JS, Weiss EG, Nogueras JJ, Wexner SD. Endorectal advancement flap in perianal Crohn's disease. Am Surg. 1998;64(2):147.
36. Mizrahi N, Wexner SD, Zmora O, Giovanna Da Silva M, Efron J, Weiss EG, et al. Endorectal advancement flap. Dis Colon Rectum. 2002;45(12):1616–21.
37. Robertson WG, Mangione JS. Cutaneous advancement flap closure. Dis Colon Rectum. 1998;41(7):884–6.
38. Sungurtekin U, Sungurtekin H, Kabay B, Tekin K, Aytekin F, Erdem E, et al. Anocutaneous VY advance-

ment flap for the treatment of complex perianal fistula. Dis Colon Rectum. 2004;47(12):2178–83.
39. Zimmerman DD, Briel JW, Gosselink MP, Schouten WR. Anocutaneous advancement flap repair of transsphincteric fistulas. Dis Colon Rectum. 2001;44(10):1474–7.
40. Jun SH, Choi GS. Anocutaneous advancement flap closure of high anal fistulas. Br J Surg. 1999;86:490–2.
41. Rojanasakul A. LIFT procedure: a simplified technique for fistula-in-ano. Tech Coloproctol. 2009;13(3):237–40.
42. Yassin N, Hammond T, Lunniss P, Phillips R. Ligation of the intersphincteric fistula tract in the management of anal fistula. A systematic review. Color Dis. 2013;15(5):527–35.
43. Vergara-Fernandez O, Espino-Urbina LA. Ligation of intersphincteric fistula tract: what is the evidence in a review? World J Gastroenterol. 2013;19:6805–13.
44. Hong KD, Kang S, Kalaskar S, Wexner SD. Ligation of intersphincteric fistula tract (LIFT) to treat anal fistula: systematic review and meta-analysis. Tech Coloproctol. 2014;18:685–91.
45. Tan KK, Tan IJ, Lim FS, Koh DC, Tsang CB. The anatomy of failures following the ligation of intersphincteric tract technique for anal fistula: a review of 93 patients over 4 years. Dis Colon Rectum. 2011;54:1368–72.
46. van Onkelen RS, Gosselink MP, Schouten WR. Ligation of the intersphincteric fistula tract in low transsphincteric fistulae: a new technique to avoid fistulotomy. Color Dis. 2013;15:587–91.
47. Hammond T, Grahn M, Lunniss P. Fibrin glue in the management of anal fistulae. Color Dis. 2004;6(5):308–19.
48. Loungnarath R, Dietz DW, Mutch MG, Birnbaum EH, Kodner IJ, Fleshman JW. Fibrin glue treatment of complex anal fistulas has low success rate. Dis Colon Rectum. 2004;47(4):432–6.
49. Singer M, Cintron J, Nelson R, Orsay C, Bastawrous A, Pearl R, Sone J, Abcarian H. Treatment of fistulas-in-ano with fibrin sealant in combination with intra-adhesive antibiotics and/or surgical closure of the internal fistula opening. Dis Colon Rectum. 2005;48:799–808.
50. Swinscoe MT, Ventakasubramaniam AK, Jayne DG. Fibrin glue for fistula-in-ano: the evidence reviewed. Tech Coloproctol. 2005;9:89–94.
51. Johnson EK, Gaw JU, Armstrong DN. Efficacy of anal fistula plug vs. fibrin glue in closure of anorectal fistulas. Dis Colon Rectum. 2006;49:371–6.
52. McGee MF, Champagne BJ, Stulberg JJ, Reynolds H, Marderstein E, Delaney CP. Tract length predicts successful closure with anal fistula plug in cryptoglandular fistulas. Dis Colon Rectum. 2010;53:1116–20.
53. Cintron JR, Abcarian H, Chaudhry V, Singer M, Hunt S, Birnbaum E, Mutch MG, Fleshman J. Treatment of fistula-in-ano using a porcine small intestinal submucosa anal fistula plug. Tech Coloproctol. 2013;17:187–91.
54. Festen C, Van Harten H. Perianal abscess and fistula-in-ano in infants. J Pediatr Surg. 1998;33(5):711–3.
55. Al-Salem AH, Laing W, Talwalker V. Fistula-in-ano in infancy and childhood. J Pediatr Surg. 1994;29(3):436–8.
56. Afşarlar ÇE, Karaman A, Tanır G, Karaman İ, Yılmaz E, Erdoğan D, et al. Perianal abscess and fistula-in-ano in children: clinical characteristic, management and outcome. Pediatr Surg Int. 2011;27(10):1063.
57. Serour F, Somekh E, Gorenstein A. Perianal abscess and fistula-in-ano in infants: a different entity? Dis Colon Rectum. 2005;48(2):359–64.
58. Poenaru D, Yazbeck S. Anal fistula in infants: etiology, features, management. J Pediatr Surg. 1993;28:1194–5.
59. Scott HJ, Northover JM. Evaluation of surgery for perianal Crohn's fistulas. Dis Colon Rectum. 1996;39:1039–43.
60. Michelassi F, Melis M, Rubin M, Hurst RD. Surgical treatment of anorectal complications in Crohn's disease. Surgery. 2000;128:597–603.
61. Makowiec F, Jehle EC, Becker HD. Starlinger Perianal abscess in Crohn's disease. Dis Colon Rectum. 1997;40:443–50.
62. de Groof EJ, Sahami S, Lucas C, Ponsioen CY, Bemelman WA, Buskens CJ. Treatment of perianal fistula in Crohn's disease: a systematic review and meta-analysis comparing seton drainage and anti-tumour necrosis factor treatment. Color Dis. 2016;18:667–75.
63. García-Olmo D, García-Arranz M, Herreros D, Pascual I, Peiro C, Rodríguez-Montes JA. A phase I clinical trial of the treatment of Crohn's fistula by adipose mesenchymal stem cell transplantation. Dis Colon Rectum. 2005;48(7):1416–23.
64. Garcia-Olmo D, Herreros D, Pascual I, Pascual JA, Del-Valle E, Zorrilla J, et al. Expanded adipose-derived stem cells for the treatment of complex perianal fistula: a phase II clinical trial. Dis Colon Rectum. 2009;52(1):79–86.

Rectovaginal Fistula

10

Jeong Eun Lee

10.1 Introduction

Rectovaginal fistula is referring to abnormal fistula tract between the rectum and vagina, and symptoms vary with the location and size of fistula. It can cause not only pain but also shame and anxiety. In the case of gas or stool leaks into the vagina, low self-esteem and restriction in expressing intimacy and interaction cause burden in the patient's social life. It can be classified by the location of fistula, low, mid, or high, or can be classified by the cause of disease. There can be various causes for rectovaginal fistula, but the most common cause is from the birth injury, and the secondary cause from underlying diseases can be from the past surgery, wound, and inflammatory bowel disease. But also, the cause can differ to the hospital level [1].

10.2 Etiology

Birth injury is the most common cause of rectovaginal fistula; it can occur with improper suture after the fourth-degree perineal lacerations or with inflammation or rupture of the wound, 7–10 days after the suture [2]. Among the inflammatory bowel diseases, rectovaginal fistula can occur mainly in Crohn's disease, and it is known to occur in 10% of women patients with Crohn's disease [2]. Cancer from the anorectal or genital organs can cause fistula between the rectum and vagina, and also pelvic irradiation can cause rectovaginal fistula, which usually occurs from 6 months to 2 years after radiation [3]. If there is bleeding through the rectum, unhealed ulceration, or newly developed anorectal pain, then rectovaginal fistula can be suspected. As symptoms can be similar to a recurrent cancer, recurrent of tumor must be distinguished. All anorectal surgeries performed in women can cause rectovaginal fistula. It is easy to occur, especially after the vaginal hysterectomy, rectocele surgery, hemorrhoidectomy, local excision of rectal tumor, and low anterior resection surgery. It also can occur from the patients with history of hysterectomy having diverticulitis or from the infection caused by inflammation, tuberculosis, or parasites originating from anal gland.

10.3 Diagnosis

In some cases, there is no subjective symptom with rectovaginal fistula, but in most cases, symptoms are gas and fecal discharge through vagina. Detailed history taking is most important as initial step. History of difficulty in birth; history of anorectal surgery, inflammatory bowel disease, and malignant tumors in anorectal or pelvic region; and history of radiation treatment should all be checked. In order to distinguish the cause

J. E. Lee (✉)
Colorectal Division, Department of Surgery,
Hansol Hospital, Seoul, South Korea
e-mail: cybexgirl@hanmail.net

D. K. Lee (ed.), *Practices of Anorectal Surgery*, https://doi.org/10.1007/978-981-13-1447-6_10

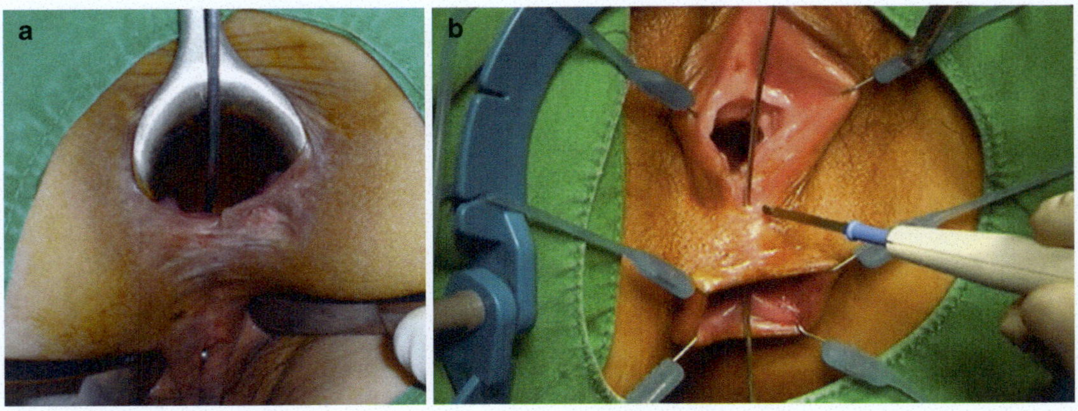

Fig. 10.1 Rectovaginal fistula. (**a**) In jackknife position, the rectovaginal fistula is checked using the probe. (**b**) In lithotomy position, Lone Star retractor is applied to secure a field of view and to identify fistula opening

of disease, symptoms like diarrhea, anal bleeding, and whether there is mucosa discharge to the anus should be checked. About 75% can be diagnosed by digital rectal examination and physical examination. The normality of perineal thickness, rupture of sphincter, and operation scar should also be examined, and anal function should also be checked [4]. Use proctoscopy and vaginal speculum to check fistula opening and condition of mucosa (Fig. 10.1). If fistula is not identified, put water into the vagina and inject air through endoscope into the rectum and check for leak of air bubbles into the vagina, or insert tampon into the vagina and inject methylene blue into the rectum and check for stain of tampon after 10 to15 minutes [5].

In the case of fistula not identified by physical examination, contrast medium should be used to check for fistula tract in the high rectovaginal fistula. Colon study or colonography with water-soluble contrast medium can be used for examination, and CT scan of the abdomen with gastrointestinal contrast material ingestion may show the contrast on the vagina [6]. In the case of birth injury, high incidence of 25% is accompanied with incontinence [7, 8], and in cases of other causes, sphincter function is an important factor in the selection of operation method; therefore, anal function tests such as anal ultrasonography, anal manometry, and compliance test for rectal capacity should be performed together. Pudendal nerve terminal motor latency test can be performed for neurophysiologic examination, but it is not typically required. It is difficult to treat rectovaginal fistula occurred from complication of radiation treatment, and it is important to distinguish the symptoms from that of the recurrent cancer. CT scan using contrast medium can help in diagnosing rectovaginal fistula caused by pelvic disease, but it is difficult to distinguish small fistula. MRI scan can also be useful for the rectovaginal fistula caused by other pelvic diseases and generally used for high type [9]. Endoscopy should be performed to examine radiation damage in the rectum, and, if necessary, biopsy of fistula should be performed under anesthesia to differentiate recurrence of cancer.

10.4 Treatment

10.4.1 Conservative Treatment

Successful treatment of rectovaginal fistula depends greatly on the cause, especially when developed from Crohn's disease or radiation injury, the prognosis is poor. In case of rectovaginal fistula due to birth injuries, it is common to wait for 6 months for natural healing, and about 50% is spontaneously healed [4, 10, 11]. Treatment for rectovaginal fistula from Crohn's disease can vary from the activity degree and invasion degree. For asymptomatic patients, specific operative treatment may not be necessary, and for symptomatic patients, staged approach should be performed to preferentially treat Crohn's disease with medical treatment and apply seton for drainage treatment of local infection [12–14]. If the local infection is cured after an active treatment of Crohn's disease, the seton is removed, and spontaneous healing of fistula can be expected [15, 16]. In the case of rectovaginal fistula from infection or malignant tumor in the anorectal or genital organs, it is important to treat after the identification of the cause of disease. Fibrin glue or fistula plug treatment for rectovaginal fistula is no longer used due to very low successful rate [12, 13].

10.4.2 Operative Treatment

In most rectovaginal fistula, surgery is the main treatment. To increase success rate, surgical method should be selected depending on the RVF location, cause, degree of infection on the surrounding tissue, history of treatment, and sphincter function [5–7]. Simple fistula in low type can be treated with local repair, and for high type, transabdominal surgery may be necessary. RVF caused by birth injury, which is the most common case, is mainly low type, and surgery can be done transperineal, transanal, and transvaginal. Surgical method can be selected based on sphincter condition, recurrence or not, and surgeon's experience, and it is essential to evaluate adequately the function of sphincter prior to the operation [10, 17]. In any surgical method, surrounding tissue should be healthy and without any inflammation or infection. From the evening before the surgery, PEG solution is administered for bowel preparation, and intravenous antibiotic is injected prior to the surgery. Insert Foley catheter just before the surgery or after anesthesia to have the patient bed rest for 2 days after the surgery. Local procedure is generally performed under spinal anesthesia, and it is not necessary to perform fecal diversion if it is not a recurrent RVF.

10.4.2.1 Transanal Approach

Transanal approach has been slightly changed from Rothenberger's (1982); however it is almost the same [18]. Local repair or advancement flap operation is adequate surgical method for low-type RVF without sphincter damage or incontinence. Fistula opening in the anus can be the consistent cause of infection, and with pressure being high in the anus, transanal approach has advantage of direct access to the opening of the anus where the pressure is high. But the surgical view is not as great as the transvaginal approach. The success rate is around 70–80% [10, 17, 19], but in the case of recurrent RVF, the rate is lower [10, 20–22]. It is not usual to consider fecal diversion prior to the operation. Main causes of failure are flap retraction and flap necrosis. Therefore, it is important to design flap including the inner circular muscle and have sufficient dissection and have the width of base of flap be twice that of the apex for smooth blood circulation. Local suture method requires sufficient dissection of surrounding tissue to reduce tension during suturing and, overlap suture the rectum and vaginal suture line to strengthen the suture area. In some advancement flap operation, it is reported to have incontinence [19, 23], but this is affected by the condition of sphincter prior to the surgery. Therefore it is important to examine sphincter function through anal physiology test prior to the surgery. The success rate of advancement flap operation when done primarily is high as 88–95% [24, 25], but in the case of recurrent surgery, the rate is lower [10].

Step 1 After spinal anesthesia, the patient is placed in jackknife position, and the rectum, vagina, and surrounding tissues are sterilized. Use Lone Star retractor to identify fistula opening and have better surgical field (Fig. 10.1).

Step 2 Incise about 1/3–1/2 of the diameter of the anal canal from the dentate line, and then use electric cautery to make flap including the mucosa, submucosa, and inner circular muscle. To decrease bleeding and dissect easily, epinephrine mixed with distilled water can be injected. The length of flap is usually 4 ~ 5 cm, the width of base is twice the size of the apex, and sufficient dissection of the base for the flap to completely cover the fistula without tension is necessary. Incise the apex with fistula opening to cover completely the RVF without tension.

Step 3 After circumferential incision is made around the entrance of fistula from the side of the rectum, hold with Allis clamp and dissect into rectovaginal septum and incise fistula tract. The defect between the rectal wall and the posterior vaginal wall is simply sutured two times with 3–0 monofilament absorbable suture thread. After hemostasis, the flap is pulled toward the anus and simply sutured on the inner sphincter muscle. The vaginal opening is not sutured and left for drainage (Fig. 10.2).

10.4.2.2 Transperineal Approach

The skin incision is made in the perineum, along the fistula between the rectum and the vagina. The incision is replaced with fourth-degree perineal laceration, and the fistula tract is completely excised, and layers are sutured with a layer-by-layer suture. Advantage is that levatorplasty, sphincteroplasty, and perineoplasty can

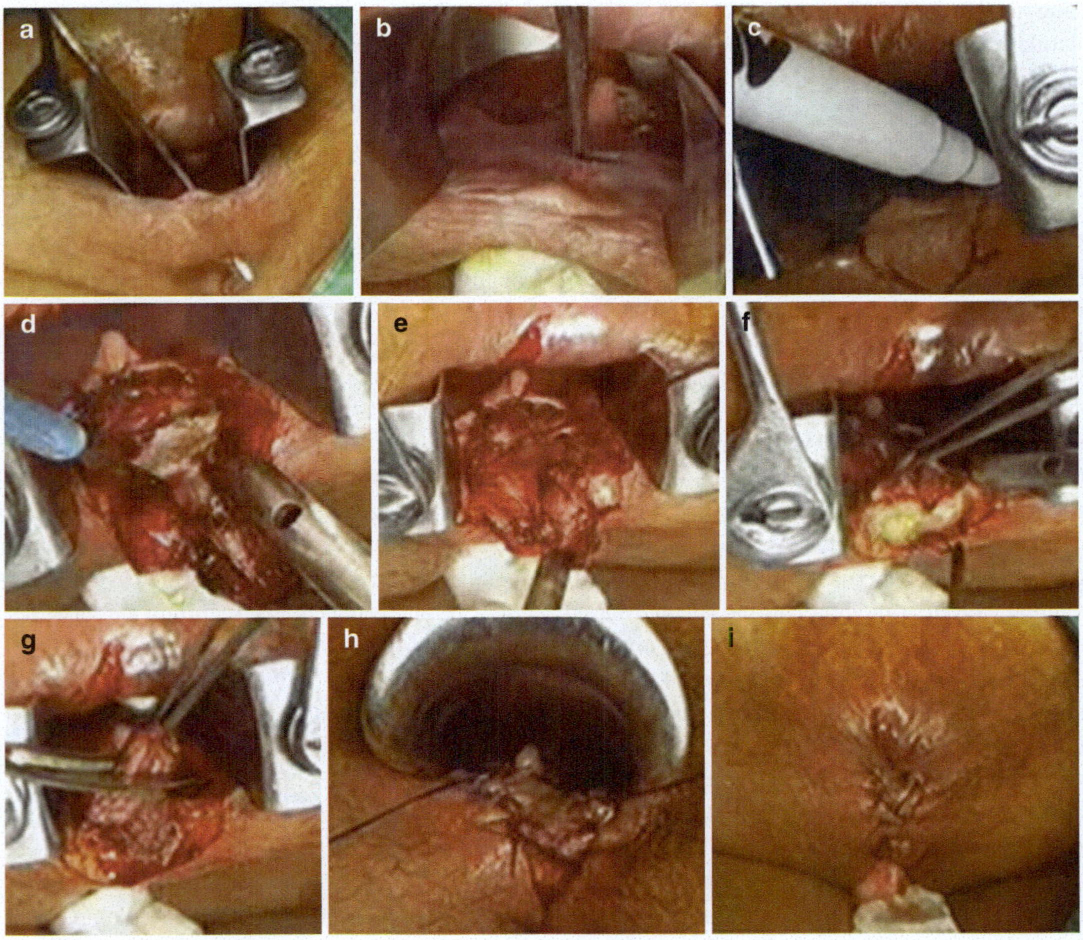

Fig. 10.2 Transanal advancement flap for rectovaginal fistula. (**a**) In jackknife position, the rectovaginal fistula is checked using the probe. (**b**) An incision is made in the anus part of the fistula opening. (**c**) An incision is made about 1/3–1/2 of the diameter of anal canal from the dentate line. (**d**) The flap is dissected including mucosa, submucosa layer, and inner circular muscle. (**e**) Circumferential incision is made around the fistula opening. (**f**) The fistula is held with Allis clamp and is dissected into vaginal wall. (**g**) The fistula is completely removed. (**h**) After suturing the rectal wall, the flap is pulled toward the anus and sutured to the internal sphincter. (**i**) The vaginal opening is not sutured and left for drainage

all be performed together and with high success rate 85–100% [26–29]. This method can also be performed on the patients with history of failure in transanal or transvaginal approach.

Step 1 After spinal anesthesia, the patient is placed in lithotomy position, and the rectum, vagina, and surrounding tissues are sterilized.

Step 2 A cross or a curved incision is made in the perineum, and rectovaginal septum is dissected until the fistula tract appears. Mucosa layer of the rectum and vagina is fully dissected from the perineal sphincter muscle and rectovaginal septum to ensure the sufficient mobility.

Step 3 Mucosa of the rectum and vagina is sutured with absorbable thread. When suturing the anal sphincter and perineal muscle, overlapping suture is recommended, and drain tube is placed in the incision site of the perineum (Fig. 10.2).

10.4.2.3 Transvaginal Approach

It is similar to transanal approach, but it has better view as it dissects the fistula from the vagina. In colorectal surgeon, as transvaginal surgery is not familiar procedure, it is not much performed. It however has the advantage in performing local repair on the patients with Crohn's disease as it is approached from the vagina which is healthy tissue, not exposed to disease. In rectovaginal fistula after irradiation, simple fistula is usually attempted with local repair, and it is better to approach from the vagina than the anus as the vagina is less irradiated [30, 31].

Step 1 After spinal anesthesia, the patient is placed in lithotomy position, and the rectum, vagina, and surrounding tissues are sterilized.

Step 2 When fistula opening is identified on the vaginal side, then incision is made from fistula opening around the posterior vaginal wall, and dissected along the rectovaginal septum, and completely excised the tract. Epinephrine mixed with distilled water is injected in the submucosa layer to reduce bleeding and to identify the margin of dissection easily.

Step 3 Vaginal wall is fully dissected from rectovaginal septum, and the rectovaginal septum and the vaginal wall are purse-string sutured orderly, so the suture surface is facing the rectum. Sufficiently dissect the side of rectovaginal septum and pull bulbospongiosus muscle and suture to reinforce the space between the rectum and the vagina, which can also have the efficacy of levatorplasty (Fig. 10.3).

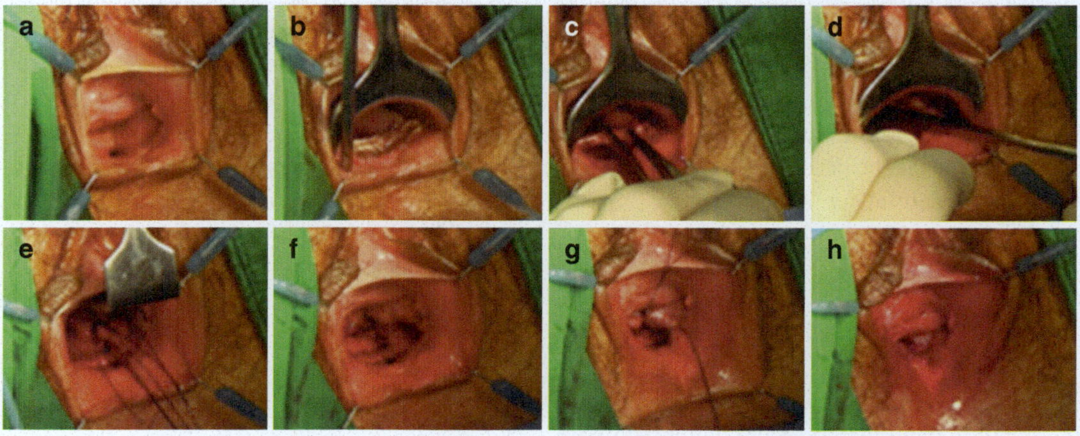

Fig. 10.3 Transvaginal approach for rectovaginal fistula. (**a**) In lithotomy position, Lone Star retractor is placed on the vagina to check the fistula opening. (**b**) An incision is made from fistula opening around the posterior vaginal wall. (**c**) The fistula is dissected along the rectovaginal septum. (**d**) The fistula is completely removed. (**e**) The rectovaginal septum is purse-string sutured. (**f**) The side of rectovaginal septum is sufficiently dissected. (**g**) The bulbospongiosus muscle is pulled and sutured. (**h**) The vaginal wall is sutured

After operation, it is recommended to maintain supine position for 4 hours until recovered from spinal anesthesia. Absolute bed rest is recommended even after restored from anesthesia. Start fluid dietary from the evening, opioids or loperamide is administered for 2 days to restrain the bowel movement, and then after, stool softener is used to prevent constipation. From the day after surgery, daily activity is possible, and Foley catheter can be removed if the patient starts walking. For the 3 days after surgery, prophylactic oral antibiotics are administered. In transvaginal approach, betadine suppository is used for the vaginal dressing.

10.5 RVF in Special Cases

10.5.1 RVF in Crohn's Disease

In the treatment of RVF in Crohn's disease, not only the location of fistula, degree of sphincter injury, and degree of inflammation around fistula are the important factors but also the main determining factor for treatment method is the activity of Crohn's disease. In active Crohn's disease, only incision and drainage should be performed like the active abscess, and medical treatment for Crohn's disease should be performed. In recent studies using infliximab, there is a report that fistula has improved up to 60%, but there are not many studies on RVF [20, 32, 33]. In patients with low-type RVF in Crohn's disease which did not involve the rectum, then rectal advancement flap operation can be performed, and fecal diversion can be helpful for wound healing [15, 31, 34, 35].

10.5.2 RVF in Radiation Injury

In the treatment of rectovaginal fistula after irradiation, it is important to secure uninjured tissue to increase success rate of the operation. Also, combining muscle replacement with healthy muscle which was not exposed to radiation with sufficient blood supply would increase success rate of the operation. Bulbocavernosus muscle replacement surgery can be performed without wide incision [36, 37], and in the case of large fistula, gracilis muscle transposition surgery can be performed, but the incidence of complication is high [38, 39].

There is controversy in performing fecal diversion in RVF surgery, and in general, it is not performed in the primary operation [35], but fecal diversion can increase the success rate in the case with RVF after irradiation or Crohn's disease or muscle transposition surgery and in the recurrent case. In many cases of the RVF of Crohn's disease, fecal diversion may stay permanent or total proctectomy needed as fistula opening is not healed after surgical correction [33, 40]. In high-type RVF, it is difficult to perform transanal or transvaginal approach; therefore transabdominal approach has to be performed, which we will not be handling in this chapter.

10.6 Summary

In rectovaginal fistula treatment, operation method should be selected considering the location and cause of fistula and condition of sphincter. Prior to the curative surgery, inflammation of the perineum around the fistula should be completely removed. For RVF after birth injury, function of sphincter should be checked through anal function test. For RVF in Crohn's disease, prior to the operative treatment, medical treatment should be performed to stabilize Crohn's disease. During the surgery, if there is not much muscle for reinforcement, the bulbospongiosus or gracilis muscle transposition should also be considered. Also prior to the complex transvaginal operation, fecal diversion should be considered.

References

1. Saclarides TJ. Rectovaginal fistula. Surg Clin North Am. 2002;82:1261–72.
2. Venkatesh KS, Ramanujam PS, Larson DM, Haywood MA. Anorectal complications of vaginal delivery. Dis Colon Rectum. 1989;32:1039–41.

3. Radcliffe AG, Ritchie JK, Hawley PR, Lennard-Jones JE, Northover JM. Anovaginal and rectovaginal fistulas in Crohn's disease. Dis Colon Rectum. 1988;31(2):94–9.
4. Goldberg SM, Gordon PM, Nivastvongs S. Essentials of anorectal surgery. Philadelphia and Toronto: KB Lippincott Company; 1980. p. 316.
5. Baig MK, Zhao RH, Yuen CH, Nogueras JJ, Singh JJ, Weiss EG, Wexner SD. Simple rectovaginal fistulas. Int J Color Dis. 2000;15:323–7.
6. Beck DE, Roberts PL, Saclarides TJ, Senagore AJ, Stamos KN, Seds W. The ASCRS textbook of colon and rectal surgery. 2nd ed. New York: Springer; 2011. p. 245–60.
7. Das B, Snyder M. Rectovaginal Fistulae. Clin Colon Rectal Surg. 2016;29:50–6.
8. Wise WE, Aguilar PS, Padmanabtan A, et al. Surgical treatment of low rectal vaginal fistulas. Dis Colon Rectum. 1991;34:271–41.
9. Ozuner G, Hull TL, Cartmill J, Fazio VW. Long-term analysis of the use of transanal rectal advancement flaps for complicated anorectal/vaginal fistulas. Dis Colon Rectum. 1996;39:10–4.
10. Lowry AC, Thorson AG, Rothenberger DA, Goldberg SA. Repair of simple rectovaginal fistulas: influence of previous repairs. Dis Colon Rectum. 1983;31:676–8.
11. Kniery K, Johnson EK, Steele SR. How I do it: Martius flap for rectovaginal fistulas. J Gastrointest Surg. 2015;19:570–4.
12. Russell TR, Gallagher DM. Low rectovaginal fistulas. Approach and treatment. Am J Surg. 1977;134:13–8.
13. White AJ, Buchsbaum HJ, Blythe JG, Lifshitz S. Use of the bulbocavernosus muscle (Martius procedure) for repair of radiation-induced rectovaginal fistulas. Obstet Gynecol. 1982;60:114–8.
14. Wexner SD, Ruiz DE, Genua J, Nogueras JJ, Weiss EG, Zmora O. Gracilis muscle interposition for the treatment of rectourethral, rectovaginal, and pouch-vaginal fistulas: results in 53 patients. Ann Surg. 2008;248:39–43.
15. de Parades V, Far HS, Etienney I, Zeitoun JD, Atienza P, Bauer P. Seton drainage and fibrin glue injection for complex anal fistulas. Color Dis. 2010;12:459–63.
16. Ellis CN. Outcomes after repair of rectovaginal fistulas using bioprosthetics. Dis Colon Rectum. 2008;51:1084–8.
17. Homsi R, Daikoku NH, Littlejohn J, Wheeless CR Jr. Episiotomy: risks of dehiscence and rectovaginal fistula. Obstet Gynecol Surv. 1994;49:803–8.
18. Tsang CBS, Madoff RD, Wong WD, et al. Anal sphincter integrity and function influences outcome in recto vaginal fistula repair. Dis Colon Rectum. 1998;41:1141–6.
19. Sudol-Szopinska I, Jakubowski W, Szczepkowski M. Contrast-enhanced endosonography for the diagnosis of anal and anovaginal fistulas. J Clin Ultrasound. 2002;30(3):145–50.
20. Löffler T, Welsch T, Mühl S, Hinz U, Schmidt J, Kienle P. Long-term success rate after surgical treatment of anorectal and rectovaginal fistulas in Crohn's disease. Int J Color Dis. 2009;24:521–6.
21. Khanduja KS, Yamashita HJ, Wise WE Jr, et al. Delayed repair of obstetric injuries of the anorectum and vagina. A stratified surgical approach. Dis Colon Rectum. 1994;37:344–9.
22. Tancer ML, Lasser D, Rosenbleum N. Rectovaginal fistula or perineal and anal sphincter disruption or both after vaginal delivery. Surg Gynecol Obstet. 1990;171:43–6.
23. Sonada T, Hull T, Piedmonte MR, Fazio VW. Outcomes of primary repair of anorectal and rectovaginal fistulas using endorectal advancement flap. Dis Colon Rectum. 2002;45:1622–8.
24. Stoker J, Rociu E, Schouten WR, Laméris JS. Anovaginal and rectovaginal fistulas: endoluminal sonography versus endoluminal MR imaging. AJR Am J Roentgenol. 2002;178:737–41.
25. Oakley SH, Brown HW, Yurteri-Kaplan L, Greer JA, Richardson ML, Adelowo A, Lindo FM, Greene KA, Fok CS, Book NM, Saiz CM, Plowright LN, Harvie HS, Pauls RN. Practice patterns regarding management of rectovaginal fistulae: a multicenter review from the Fellows' Pelvic Research Network. Female Pelvic Med Reconstr Surg. 2015;21:123–8.
26. Corte H, Maggiori L, Treton X, Lefevre JH, Ferron M, Panis Y. Rectovaginal fistula: what is the optimal strategy?: an analysis of 79 patients undergoing 286 procedures. Ann Surg. 2015;262:855–60.
27. Wiskind AK, Thompson JD. Transverse transperineal repair of rectovaginal fistulas in the lower vagina. Am J Obstet Gynecol. 1992;167:694–9.
28. Fürst A, Schmidbauer C, Swol-Ben J, Iesalnieks I, Schwandner O, Agha A. Gracilis transposition for repair of recurrent anovaginal and rectovaginal fistulas in Crohn's disease. Int J Color Dis. 2008;23:349–53.
29. Yamamoto T. Disappointing results following proctectomy with end-colostomy for anorectal Crohn's disease. J Crohns Colitis. 2013;7(4):e150.
30. Mazier WP, Senagore AJ, Schiesel EC. Operative repair of anovaginal and rectovaginal fistulas. Dis Colon Rectum. 1995;38:4–6.
31. Rothenberger DA, Christenson CE, Balcos EG, Schottler JL, Nemer FD, Nivatvongs S, Goldberg SM. Endorectal advancement flap for treatment of simple rectovaginal fistula. Dis Colon Rectum. 1982;25:297–300.
32. Sands BE, Blank MA, Patel K, et al. Long–term treatment of rectovaginal fistula in Crohn's disease' response to infliximab in the ACCENT II Study. Clin Gastroenterol Hepatol. 2004;2:912–20.
33. MacRae HM, McLeod RS, Cohen Z, Stern H, Reznick R. Treatment of rectovaginal fistulas that has failed previous repair attempts. Dis Colon Rectum. 1995;38:921–5.
34. Pinto RA, Peterson TV, Shawki S, Davila GW, Wexner SD. Are there predictors of outcome follow-

ing rectovaginal fistula repair? Dis Colon Rectum. 2010;53:1240–7.
35. Hull TL, fazio VW. Surgical approaches to low anovagi9nal fistula in Crohn's disease. Am J Surg. 1997;173:95–8.
36. Bhome R, Monga A, Nugent KP. A transvaginal approach to rectovaginal fistulae for the colorectal surgeon; technical notes and cse series. Tech Coloproctol. 2018;22:305–11.
37. Champagne BJ, McGee MF. Rectovaginal fistula. Surg Clin N Am. 2010;90:69–82.
38. Chung CS, Lee DK, George BD, Mortensen NJ. Clinical outcome of rectovaginal fistula in Crohn's disease. J Coloproctol. 2008;23:10–5.
39. McNevin MS, Lee PY, Bax TW. Martius flap: an adjunct for repair of complex, low rectovaginal fistula. Am J Surg. 2007;193:597–9.
40. Hull TL, Bartus C, Bast J, Floruta C, Lopez R. Multimedia article. Success of episioproctotomy for cloaca and rectovaginal fistula. Dis Colon Rectum. 2007;50:97–101.

11 Rectal Prolapse

Gwanchul Lee

11.1 Introduction

Rectal prolapse happens when the entire wall of the rectum slides through the anus, affecting daily life (Fig. 11.1). It is most common in women over 60s and in the age over 50s, it is 5~6 times more in women than men [1–3]. Anatomically in rectal prolapse, diastasis of levator ani, deep cul-de-sac, elongated sigmoid colon, and mesorectum and patulous anus are seen. Also, through endoscopy, it can be accompanied by solitary rectal ulcer [4, 5] and is common to accompany incontinence or defecation disorder [6]. There are two hypotheses about the occurrence of the disease: sliding hernia (Moschowitz) and rectal intussusceptions (Broden & Snellman) [7, 8]. The former hypothesis is that the rectal wall slides down through defect of pelvic fascia. This is based on that the patients with rectal prolapse show deep rectovaginal pouch or rectovesical pouch. The rectal intussusception hypothesis is that in defecography, rectal intussusception occurs in the upper part of the pelvic floor and driven down to the anus. In any hypothesis, it is considered the same that the weakened connection between the rectal wall and the endopelvic fascia drives down to the anus. But it is not clear whether the defect of pelvic floor is caused by prolapse or it is easily driven down due to the defect.

G. Lee (✉)
Colorectal Division, Department of Surgery, Hansol Hospital, Seoul, South Korea

11.2 Examination

Symptoms of rectal prolapse in early stage start with protrusion of the rectum mucosa during bowel movement and, gradually, coughing or protrusion of the entire layer of rectum when straining in squatting position. This is different from the prolapse in hemorrhoids as the hemorrhoids protrude radially, but rectal prolapse involves the rectal mucosa concentrically protruding all of the rectum.

In most patients, they suffer from incontinence caused by prolapsed rectum which constantly loosens the sphincter muscle. The constant prolapse can constantly stimulate rectoanal inhibitory reflex and can also worsen incontinence by hypotrophied sphincter from the pudendal nerve damage [9–11]. On the other hand, some patients have constipation due to blockage in the anus from prolapsed rectum and can get worse by straining as it can bring disharmony in the pelvic floor muscle [12]. There are some cases accompanied by not only the prolapse of the rectum but also the urinary incontinence or protrusion of other pelvic organs (Fig. 11.2). In severe rectum prolapse, it can easily be diagnosed by protrusion of the rectum, but in early stage, it is hard to diagnose as it is often concealed. When straining in squatting position, it can be diagnosed by protruded rectal mucosa from the relaxation of the anal sphincter, but in the case of difficulty in examination, it can be checked by the rectal mucous that comes with

D. K. Lee (ed.), *Practices of Anorectal Surgery*, https://doi.org/10.1007/978-981-13-1447-6_11

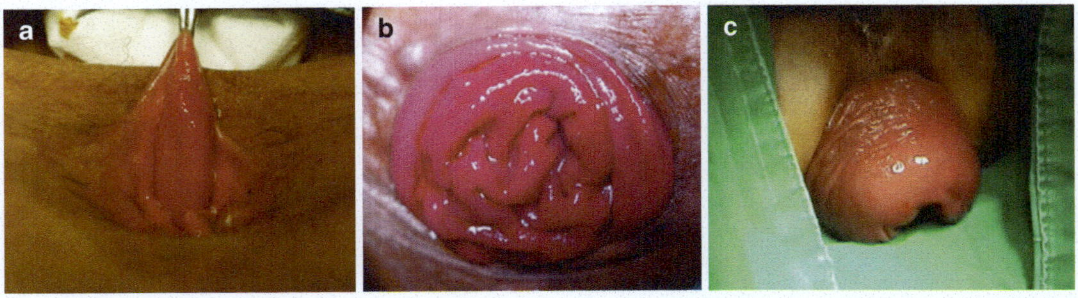

Fig. 11.1 Rectal prolapse. (**a**) Mucosal prolapse. (**b**) Incomplete rectal prolapse. (**c**) Full-thickness complete rectal prolapse

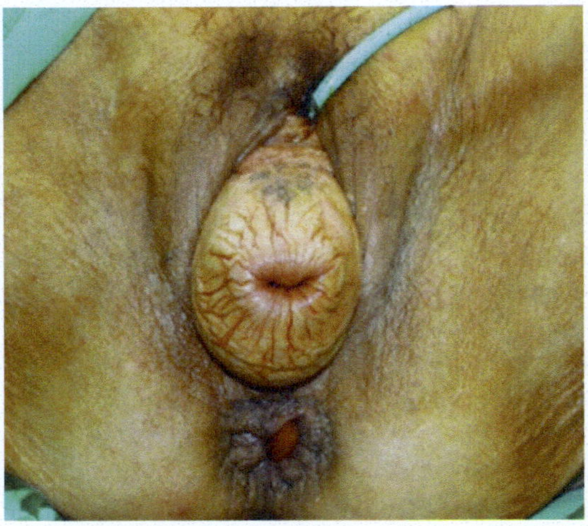

Fig. 11.2 Rectal prolapse including pelvic organ prolapse

slowly pulled gauze that was inserted into the rectum. In the case of rectal prolapse, as there can be other accompanied prolapsed organs (uterus, bladder, etc.), the accompanied symptoms should also be checked, and if detected, concomitant treatment should also be considered [13–15].

Defecography can be helpful in the early diagnosis of rectal prolapse (Fig. 11.3). Also, as it provides much information about the accompanied abnormal findings such as obtuse of anorectal angle and descending of pelvic floor, it is a very useful examination method [4, 16].

Anal ultrasonography can help distinguish the anal sphincter damage and rectal prolapse caused by rectal tumor. Anal manometry can be used for determining the degree of anal sphincter weakness to predict postoperative fecal incontinence [17, 18]. Colonoscopy can help in diagnosing the isolated ulcers of the rectum caused by rectal prolapse and rectal intussusceptions (Fig. 11.4) [19]. In addition, dynamic magnetic resonance imaging can be used to examine the presence of other pelvic organ prolapse [20].

In colonoscopy it is shown in the forms of multiple pseudopolyposis or isolated ulcers of the rectum.

11.3 Treatment

11.3.1 Non-operative Treatment

Treatment of rectal prolapse aims to cure the protruded rectum and relieve accompanied symptoms including rectal bleeding, incontinence or constipation, and incomplete defecation. Conservative treatment rarely cures, and the only method for a complete cure is surgery. But in cases when surgery is not possible, then fecal incontinence or constipation symptoms should be relieved for patient's quality of life. Improve by using fiber and stool softener. If there is difficulty in pushing back the prolapsed rectum, sprinkling sugar will reduce edema and will make it easier to return into the rectum [21]. Patients with fecal incontinence, it should be treated prior to the surgery which will help bowel control after the surgery, and if the prolapse is left untreated for long term, fecal incontinence will not be recovered [22, 23].

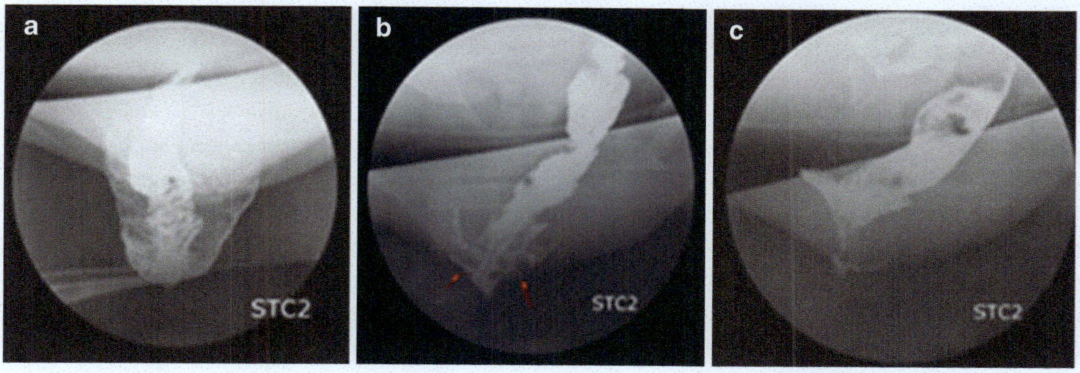

Fig. 11.3 Defecography in rectal prolapse. (**a**) Full-thickness external rectal prolapse. (**b**) Incomplete rectal prolapse. (**c**) Internal rectal intussusception

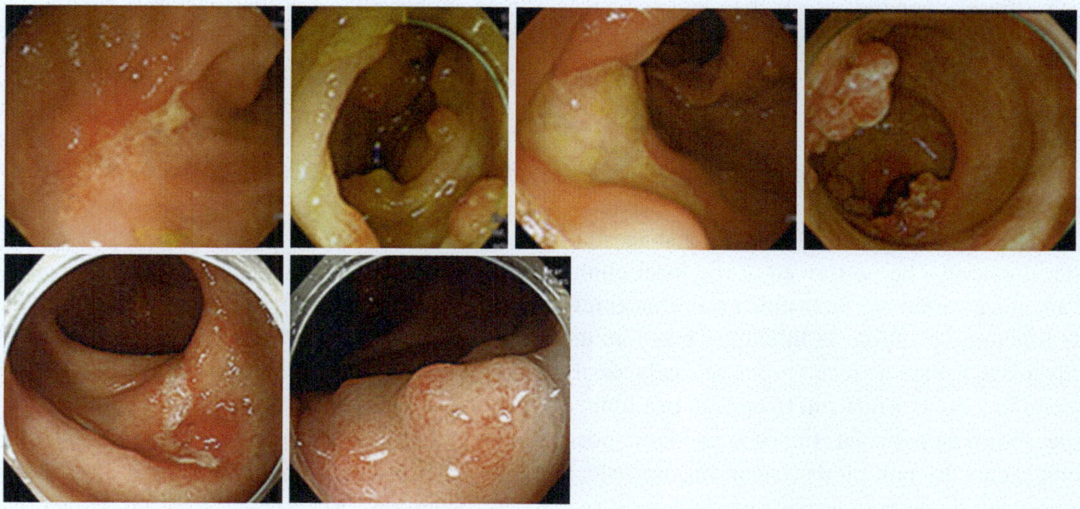

Fig. 11.4 Large variety of colonoscopic findings of solitary rectal ulcer syndrome

11.3.2 Operative Treatment

Due to the high recurrence rate, surgeons should be very cautious in selecting the operation method. When selecting the operation method, anatomical abnormalities and cause, patient's general condition, and defecation disorders like fecal incontinence or constipation should be considered. The two operation methods are transanal and transabdominal approach, and it is important to have a surgeon who is capable of both approaches. This is because, even if the other approach is more appropriate for the patient, only one method will be considered due to the capability of the surgeon. Recently, laparoscopic rectopexy can be applied to almost all the patients without severe cardiac or lung disease. Also, if accompanied with bladder or uterine prolapse, as it is more efficient to operate together, multidisciplinary approach is recommended or should have surgical technique to fix everything together. Here we would like to focus on the transanal approach.

In transanal approach, there are Delorme's operation, Altemeier's operation, Thiersch's operation, Gant-Miwa operation, and PPH for mucosal prolapse. In general, Delorme's and Altemeier's operation are commonly used [24, 25]. Delorme's operation is less invasive than Altemeier's operation, has less postoperative complications, and is more appropriate for elderly patients with comorbidity. If the length of prolapsed rectum is over 5 cm, it is better to excise to lower the recurrence rate. In young and active patients, transabdominal rectopexy with or without resection of the sigmoid colon can be used.

11.3.2.1 PPH for Mucosal Prolapse

Using the stapler for hemorrhoidectomy to incise rectal mucosa cannot be used for the complete rectal prolapse which is the prolapse of the entire rectal wall. It is the most appropriate basic treatment for hemorrhoid accompanied by rectal mucosa prolapse; however it has risk of recurrence. The operation method is similar to the hemorrhoid operation using the stapler device. However, purse-string suture in zigzag form to maximize the excision width will lower the recurrence and can excise up to 3 cm width (Fig. 11.5).

11.3.2.2 Delorme's Operation

It is relatively easy to adapt surgical procedures, and as it can be performed under spinal anesthesia, it can also be performed at the local clinic. Patient's position can be in either prone jackknife or lithotomy position. In lithotomy position, the advantage is that the rectal prolapse can be easily identified, but it is difficult to operate in a limited space with an assistant. In prone jackknife position, excise by pulling the rectal mucosa, which will make it easier to remove the prolapsed rectum sufficiently; therefore we use this position in our clinic.

Surgery is performed in a circumferential incision of the mucosa using an electrocautery around 1.5 cm above the dentate line, and then dissect the mucosa and separate from the muscle layer of the rectum then dissect until the proximal is no longer extended. To facilitate dissection and reduce bleeding, epinephrine mixed with normal saline can be injected; however, in our hospital, it is only used to distinguish the mucosa from the muscle layer at the first incision, and it is no longer used during dissection. The mucosal layer of the rectum is dissected until it is no longer pulled, and the muscles are folded vertically in four directions to form plication, and then additional 8 points in between. The plication suture is done by pushing the muscle layer into the anal canal. The mucosal layer can be sutured together with plication, or plicate only the muscle layer, and suture can be done separately (Fig. 11.6). As this approach has almost no postoperative complications, it is the preferred method for patients with poor condition, but it can result in postoperative tenesmus and cause heavy feeling. Also, patients with severe constipation should consider a different surgical method, as it can be the cause for early recurrence of straining in defecation after surgery. In the case of long-term prolapse, it can be possible that the damaged sphincter cannot recover even after the surgery, and incontinence is likely to persist with patulous anus, so in this case, Thiersch's procedure is combined using lapa-tape. This procedure is mostly used in prolapse within 5 cm, and as it is generally considered safe, it has been used for patients with poor general condition. Recurrence rate (10–15%) is known to be higher than the Trans-abdominal approach but this might be coming from the difference in the selected patients [26–28]. Which means, as this is mostly used in the elderly patients and therefore the recurrence rate can be higher, but in the other patients the recurrence rate is known to be no different [29].

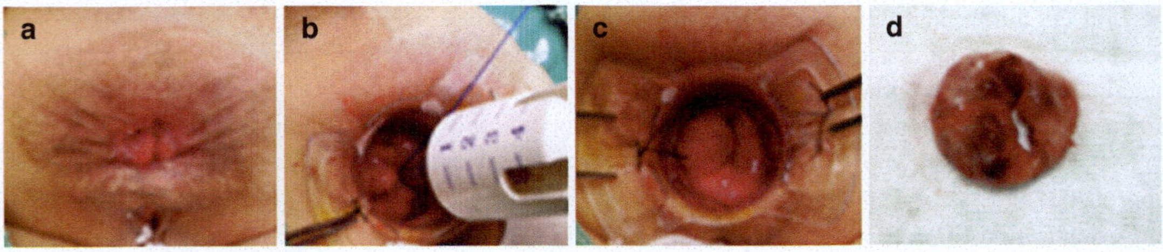

Fig. 11.5 Stapled transanal rectal resection (STARR). (**a**) Mucosal prolapse. (**b**) Insertion of circular stapler after purse-string suture in the lower rectum. (**c**) Anastomotic line after firing of the circular stapler. (**d**) Resected rectal mucosa after the procedure

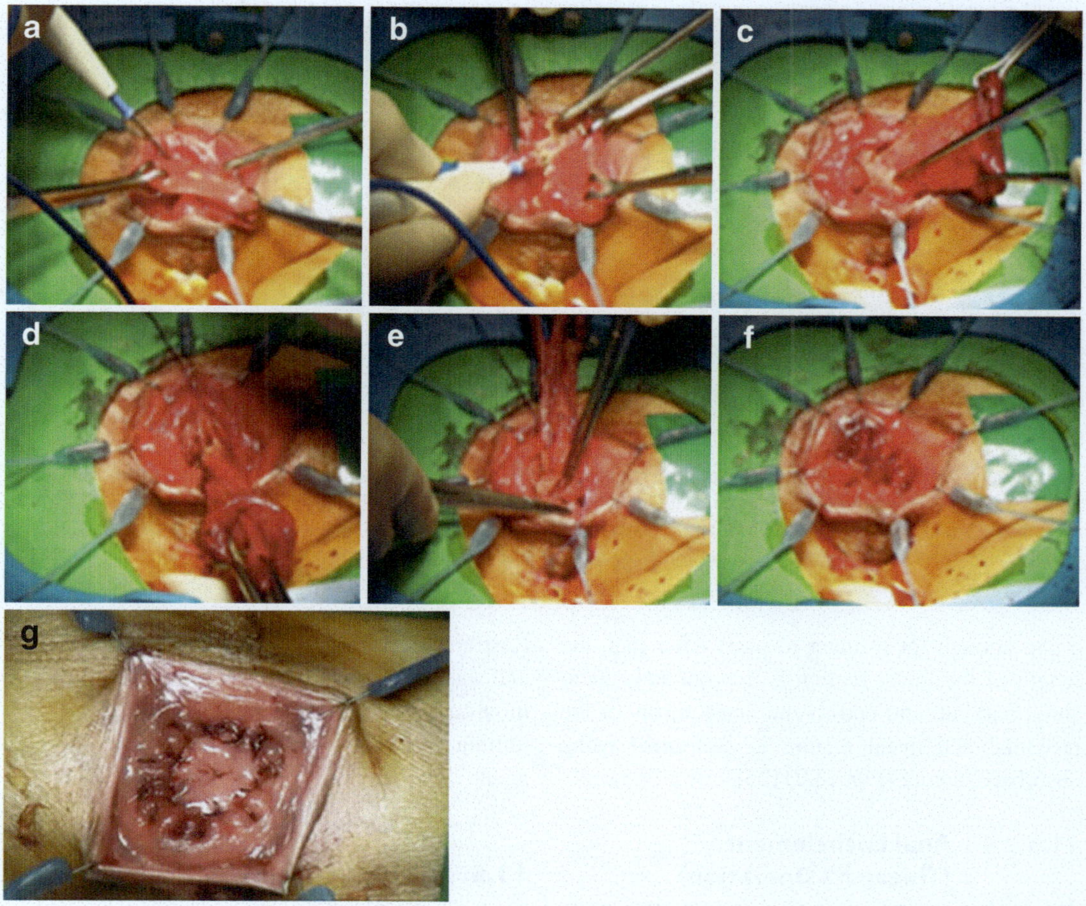

Fig. 11.6 Delorme's operation. (**a**) Jackknife position and perianal retraction via Lone Star retractor. (**b**) Incision by pulling the rectal mucosa. (**c**) Circumferential incision of rectal mucosa. (**d**) Circumferential excision by prolapsed rectal mucosa. (**e**) 4-point plication suture in resected rectal muscle. (**f**) Additional 8-point suture plication. (**g**) End of plication suture

11.3.2.3 Perineal Rectosigmoidectomy (Altemeier's Operation)

This is an operation anastomosing proximal and distal rectum after excision of the prolapsed rectum and can be combined with levatorplasty, closing the deep rectovaginal pouch or rectovesicular pouch in the anterior part during the surgery, narrowing the pelvic floor. However, even after levatorplasty, there is no significant difference in the incontinence, but the recurrence rate is known to be lower [30, 31]. Recurrence rate is known to be relatively higher than the transabdominal approach, but as there is great difference in the patient group, the actual comparison is difficult. In general, the recurrence rate within 2 years is about 15–30% [32, 33].

Surgery is performed in circumferential incision of the entire rectal wall from 2 to 3 cm above the dentate line, and then proximal incision is made. The anterior pouch of Douglas is opened, and by holding it with hand, the mesorectum of the posterior side of the rectum is dissected. The mesorectum is elongated due to long-term prolapse of the rectum, so it can be easily ligated and excised. By using Harmonic scalpel or LigaSure, it can be dissected easily without ligating the blood vessels. There is no clear standard guideline for up to which point of the proximal, but it can usually go up to the elongated upper rectum or above. Before anastomosis, the peritoneum is sutured, at this time, close the deep rectovaginal pouch or rectovesicular pouch. In addition, levatoplasty is performed by exposing the levator muscle, which is sutured with

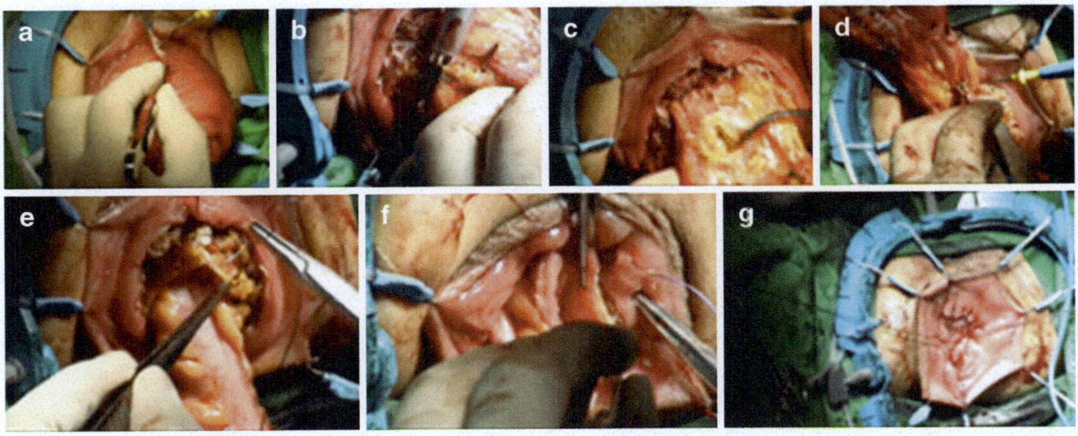

Fig. 11.7 Altemeier's operation. (**a**) Perianal retraction via Lone Star retractor and circumferential full layer incision above 2–3 cm of dentate line. (**b**) Opening the pouch of Douglas. (**c**) Dissection of mesentery and ligation. (**d**) Excision of the prolapsed rectum. (**e**) Levatorplasty done by exposing the levator muscle. (**f**) End-to-end anastomosis. (**g**) Finally suturing of rectal mucosa

a gap enough for a finger to pass. After that, the length of the lower rectum is appropriately measured and cut, and end-to-end anastomosis of the proximal and distal rectum is performed using absorbable suture (Fig. 11.7) [25].

11.3.2.4 Anal Encirclement (Thiersch's Operation)

This technique is a surgical procedure that complements the weakened sphincter tone by using nylon tape outside the internal sphincter. Surgery is performed in a prone jackknife position. Incision is made perpendicular at 6 o'clock and 12 o'clock directions 1 cm from the anal verge. Use Cleveland forceps on the incised site to pass nylon tape to both sides of outer side of the inner sphincter muscle. Ligate nylon tape penetrating 360° with enough space at the anal canal for no.9 bougie to pass. Then, the incised anal region is sutured, and the operation is completed (Fig. 11.8).

11.4 Postoperative Management

After the Delorme's operation, administer liquid diet immediately, and from the day after surgery, start sitz bath. Antibiotics should be injected before and after the operation. Prior to the Altemeier's operation, insert a Foley catheter, and inject antibiotics before and after the operation. Restrain defecation for 2–3 days after the surgery, and start sitz bath the day after surgery. It is common to have postoperative incontinence symptom, in case of which, administer an antidiarrheal agent.

11.5 Complications

11.5.1 Fecal Incontinence

Prior to surgery, if fecal incontinence is accompanied by an already weakened anal sphincter muscle, postoperative symptoms may worsen. In this case, it is necessary to combine fiber supplement and antidiarrheal agent which increase the volume of stool to avoid the loose stool. Biofeedback training can be helpful in a few cases [34]. Prior to the surgery, if there is high possibility of causing severe incontinence, combining Thiersch operation can be considered.

11.5.2 Recurrence

In general, transanal approach has higher recurrence rate than the transabdominal approach [35] (Fig. 11.9). However, when choosing the operation method, recurrence rate could be higher due to variables like patient's age and general condition.

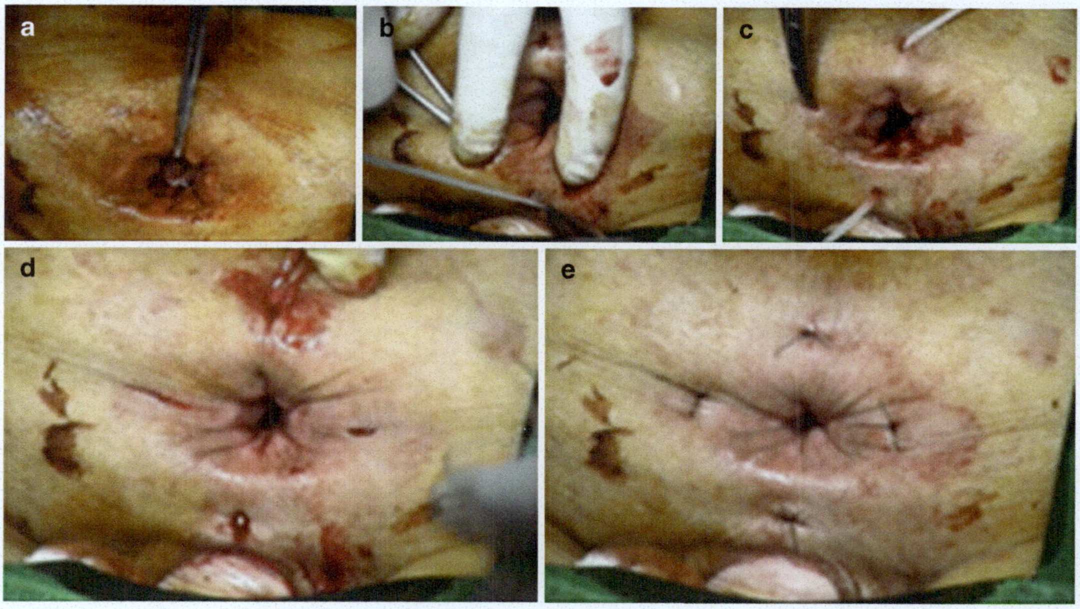

Fig. 11.8 Thiersch's operation. (**a**) Perpendicular incision at 6 and 12 o'clock. (**b**) Cleveland forceps inserted outside the inner sphincter. (**c**) Insertion of nylon tape. (**d**) Opposite site insertion of nylon tape, 360°. (**e**) Nylon tape ligated with enough space for no.9 bougie to pass

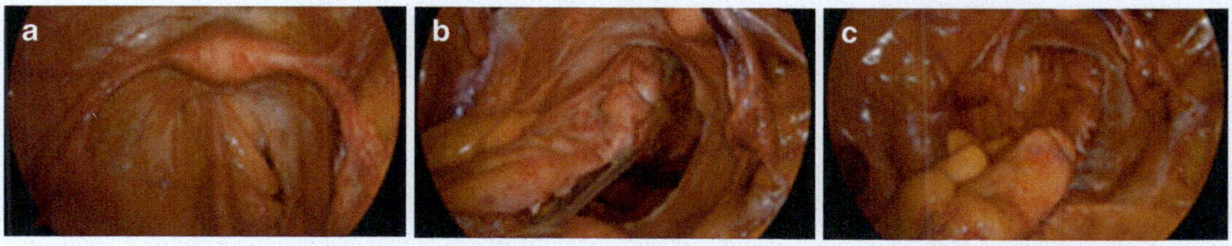

Fig. 11.9 Laparoscopic ventral rectopexy. (**a**) Pelvis inlet. (**b**) Dissection of mesorectum and application of polypropylene mesh. (**c**) Repair of dissected rectum

Therefore, give sufficient explanation on the recurrence prior to the rectal prolapse operation, and when recurred, it is important to perform surgical approach considering the operation method performed in the prior surgery. In the case of recurrent rectal prolapse, resection of the rectum has to be considered, but the surgery has to be decided after determining the degree of blood circulation in the remaining rectum [36].

11.6 Summary

Rectal prolapse is mostly seen in older patients which relates to the higher risk of surgery. It is important to apply appropriate surgical procedures for the patient considering the patient's general condition. Also, it is necessary to determine whether to resolve together the other accompanied diseases like fecal incontinence or pelvic organ prolapse. In the case of postoperative recurrence, a different surgical approach to the prior surgery should be considered.

References

1. Nygaard I, Barber MD, Burgio KL, Kenton K, Meikle S, Schaffer J, et al. Prevalence of symptomatic pelvic floor disorders in US women. JAMA. 2008;300(11):1311–6. Pubmed Central PMCID: 2918416.

2. Harmston C, Jones OM, Cunningham C, Lindsey I. The relationship between internal rectal prolapse and internal anal sphincter function. Colorectal Dis. 2011;13(7):791–5.
3. Bordeianou L, Lee KY, Rockwood T, Baxter NN, Lowry A, Mellgren A, et al. Anal resting pressures at manometry correlate with the Fecal Incontinence Severity Index and with presence of sphincter defects on ultrasound. Dis Colon Rectum. 2008;51(7):1010–4.
4. Bordeianou L, Hicks CW, Kaiser AM, Alavi K, Sudan R, Wise PE. Rectal prolapse: an overview of clinical features, diagnosis, and patient-specific management strategies. J Gastrointest Surg. 2014;18(5):1059–69.
5. Felt-Bersma RJ, Tiersma ES, Cuesta MA. Rectal prolapse, rectal intussusception, rectocele, solitary rectal ulcer syndrome, and enterocele. Gastroenterol Clin N Am. 2008;37(3):645–68, ix.
6. Dvorkin LS, Gladman MA, Epstein J, Scott SM, Williams NS, Lunniss PJ. Rectal intussusception in symptomatic patients is different from that in asymptomatic volunteers. Br J Surg. 2005;92(7):866–72.
7. Gourgiotis S, Baratsis S. Rectal prolapse. Int J Color Dis. 2007;22(3):231–43.
8. Kairaluoma MV, Kellokumpu IH. Epidemiologic aspects of complete rectal prolapse. Scand J Surg. 2005;94(3):207–10.
9. Broden B, Snellman B. Procidentia of the rectum studied with cineradiography. A contribution to the discussion of causative mechanism. Dis Colon Rectum. 1968;11(5):330–47.
10. Kaufman HS, Buller JL, Thompson JR, Pannu HK, DeMeester SL, Genadry RR, et al. Dynamic pelvic magnetic resonance imaging and cystocolpoproctography alter surgical management of pelvic floor disorders. Dis Colon Rectum. 2001;44(11):1575–83; discussion 83–4. PubMed PMID: 11711726.
11. Myers JO, Rothenberger DA. Sugar in the reduction of incarcerated prolapsed bowel. Report of two cases. Dis Colon Rectum. 1991;34(5):416–8.
12. Sun WM, Read NW, Donnelly TC, Bannister JJ, Shorthouse AJ. A common pathophysiology for full thickness rectal prolapse, anterior mucosal prolapse and solitary rectal ulcer. Br J Surg. 1989;76(3):290–5.
13. Wallenhorst T, Bouguen G, Brochard C, Cunin D, Desfourneaux V, Ropert A, Bretagne JF, Siproudhis L. Long-term impact of full-thickness rectal prolapse treatment on fecal incontinence. Surgery. 2015;158(1):104–11.
14. Cunin D, Siproudhis L, Desfourneaux V, Berkelmans I, Meunier B, Bretagne JF, Bouguen G. No surgery for full-thickness rectal prolapse: what happens with continence? World J Surg. 2013;37(6):1297–302.
15. Lindsey I. Commentary: Best practice in rectal prolapse. Colorectal Dis. 2010;12(6):512–4.
16. Altemeier WA, Culbertson WR, Schowengerdt C, Hunt J. Nineteen years' experience with the one-stage perineal repair of rectal prolapse. Ann Surg. 1971;173(6):993–1006.
17. Moschcowitz AV. The pathogenesis, anatomy and cure of prolapse of the rectum. Surg Gynecol Obstet. 1912;15:7–21.
18. Glasgow SC, Birnbaum EH, Kodner IJ, Fleshman JW, Dietz DW. Preoperative anal manometry predicts continence after perineal proctectomy for rectal prolapse. Dis Colon Rectum. 2006;49(7):1052–8.
19. Snooks SJ, Henry MM, Swash M. Anorectal incontinence and rectal prolapse: differential assessment of the innervation to puborectalis and external anal sphincter muscles. Gut. 1985;26(5):470–6.
20. Hawkins AT, Olariu AG, Savitt LR, Gingipally S, Wakamatsu MM, Pulliam S, Weinstein MM, Bordeianou L. Impact of rising grades of internal rectal intussusception on fecal continence and symptoms of constipation. Dis Colon Rectum. 2016;59(1):54–61.
21. Lieberth M, Kondylis LA, Reilly JC, Kondylis PD. The Delorme repair for full-thickness rectal prolapse: a retrospective review. Am J Surg. 2009;197(3):418–23.
22. Senapati A, Nicholls RJ, Thomson JP, Phillips RK. Results of Delorme's procedure for rectal prolapse. Dis Colon Rectum. 1994;37(5):456–60.
23. Watkins BP, Landercasper J, Belzer GE, Rechner P, Knudson R, Bintz M, Lambert P. Long-term follow-up of the modified Delorme procedure for rectal prolapse. Arch Surg. 2003;138(5):498–502.
24. Schultz I, Mellgren A, Dolk A, Johansson C, Holmström B. Long-term results and functional outcome after Ripstein rectopexy. Dis Colon Rectum. 2000;43(1):35–43.
25. Altman D, Zetterstrom J, Schultz I, Nordenstam J, Hjern F, Lopez A, Mellgren A. Pelvic organ prolapse and urinary incontinence in women with surgically managed rectal prolapse: a population-based case-control study. Dis Colon Rectum. 2006;49(1):28–35.
26. Senapati A, Gray RG, Middleton LJ, Harding J, Hills RK, Armitage NC, Buckley L, Northover JM, PROSPER Collaborative Group. PROSPER: a randomised comparison of surgical treatments for rectal prolapse. Color Dis. 2013;15(7):858–68.
27. Habr-Gama A, Jacob CE, Jorge JM, Seid VE, Marques CF, Mantese JC, Kiss DR, Gama-Rodrigues J. Rectal procidentia treatment by perineal rectosigmoidectomy combined with levator ani repair. Hepato-Gastroenterology. 2006;53(68):213–7.
28. Chun SW, Pikarsky AJ, You SY, Gervaz P, Efron J, Weiss E, Nogueras JJ, Wexner SD. Perineal rectosigmoidectomy for rectal prolapse: role of levatorplasty. Tech Coloproctol. 2004;8(1):3–8.
29. Altomare DF, Binda G, Ganio E, De Nardi P, Giamundo P, Pescatori M. Rectal Prolapse Study Group. Long-term outcome of Altemeier's procedure for rectal prolapse. Dis Colon Rectum. 2009;52(4):698–703.
30. Riansuwan W, Hull TL, Bast J, Hammel JP, Church JM. Comparison of perineal operations with abdominal operations for full-thickness rectal prolapse. World J Surg. 2010;34(5):1116–22.

31. Khaikin M, Wexner SD. Treatment strategies in obstructed defecation and fecal incontinence. World J Gastroenterol. 2006;12(20):3168–73. Pubmed Central PMCID: 4087958.
32. Bachoo P, Brazzelli M, Grant A. Surgery for complete rectal prolapse in adults. Cochrane Database Syst Rev. 2000;(2):CD001758.
33. Tou S, Brown SR, Nelson RL. Surgery for complete (full-thickness) rectal prolapse in adults. Cochrane Database Syst Rev. 2015;(11):CD001758.
34. González-Argenté FX, Jain A, Nogueras JJ, Davila GW, Weiss EG, Wexner SD. Prevalence and severity of urinary incontinence and pelvic genital prolapse in females with anal incontinence or rectal prolapse. Dis Colon Rectum. 2001;44(7):920–6.
35. Bordeianou L, Hicks CW, Olariu A, Savitt L, Pulliam SJ, Weinstein M, Rockwood T, Sylla P, Kuo J, Wakamatsu M. Effect of coexisting pelvic floor disorders on fecal incontinence quality of life scores: a prospective, survey-based study. Dis Colon Rectum. 2015;58(11):1091–7.
36. Pescatori M, Spyrou M, Pulvirenti d'Urso A. A prospective evaluation of occult disorders in obstructed defecation using the 'iceberg diagram'. Color Dis. 2006;8(9):785–9.

12 Outlet Obstructive Constipation

Gwanchul Lee

12.1 Introduction

Many patients know that constipation is an opposite of a fecal incontinence, which is true for the patients with actual fecal incontinence, but express it as diarrhea. At this time, the expression diarrhea is only a polite expression of the loss of bowel control ability. Actually, constipation and fecal incontinence can occur together, and to understand the role of anal physiology laboratory where the patients are examined, it could be helpful to understand the normal bowel movement. A mass peristaltic wave develops in the dilated left colon with stool, and the stool descends to the rectum below the sigmoid. Once the stool enters the rectum, the external sphincter contracts and internal sphincter relaxes which is the sampling reflex and also bowel control mechanism starts. Once the rectal compliance occurs, initial stimulus to defecate is delivered to the intrarectal pressure causing decrease in resting pressure of the anal canal and voluntary contraction of the external sphincter which result in defecation [1, 2].

When the bowel movement occurs at a generally acceptable time and place or the rectal compliance is reached its limitation, and no longer affordable to restrain defecation, then the natural bowel movement occurs. In defecation process, with normal relaxation of the anorectal angle and intentionally increased abdominal pressure by Valsalva manuever results the increase in the rectal pressure, then the relaxation and contraction of the internal and external anal sphincter occur. At this time, normal pelvic descent occurs to a certain degree. When an additional peristaltic wave is generated, the contents in left colon are completely emptied [3, 4]. If this does not occur, bowel movement will break out for the next 24 hours. After defecation, anal pressure, abdominal pressure, and anorectal angle return to normal status. Within this process, if one of the parts have disorder or blocked, then outlet obstructive constipation occurs. Outlet obstructive constipations occur in the cases with non-relaxing puborectalis syndrome, abnormal high anal pressure, extreme compliance of the rectum, constipation from external compression of the rectum, incomplete defecation, rectal intussusceptions, and with severe descend of pelvic floor [5, 6]. It is difficult to distinguish whether the pelvic descent or other rectocele occurrence is due to excessive force from outlet obstruction of other causes or it could be the primary cause of outlet obstruction. However, it is proper to see it as secondary changes from constipation. In this chapter, we will only deal with non-relaxing puborectalis syndrome and rectocele out of all the causes of the outlet obstructive constipation.

G. Lee (✉)
Colorectal Division, Department of Surgery, Hansol Hospital, Seoul, South Korea

D. K. Lee (ed.), *Practices of Anorectal Surgery*, https://doi.org/10.1007/978-981-13-1447-6_12

12.2 Examination

In the first examination of the patients with constipation or fecal incontinence, whether to perform basic anorectal physiology laboratory test can differ from doctors. However, in general, when a patient over 50 years is suffering from pelvic floor dysfunction and has no experience in colonoscopy, the most important first step is to identify what the patient is really suffering from. This is because patients tend to use indirect way to express the symptoms, as they feel embarrassed and awkward in the examination room. For instance, they wet their underwear due to incontinence but express it as diarrhea. Once this first step is carefully defined and symptoms are identified, if possible, the symptoms should be quantitatively and qualitatively analyzed. For example, it is very important to know whether incontinence is with gas, water or solid stool, constipation with soft or hard stool, degree of excessive staining, difficulty in feeling bowel movement, and frequency of defecation. Once detailed history is taken, it should be determined whether additional anal function tests are necessary through the physical examination. If defect of the anterior side of the sphincter muscle is clear in the incontinence patients with multiple birth history, it may not be an indication for additional testing. In the case with fecal impaction, patients have liquid stool, which can be treated through bowel rehabilitation training rather than additional tests. In the case with acute proctitis, obstructive lesions, and obvious rectal prolapse, you can plan the treatment immediately. If the initial physical examination is not able to give clear answer, you might need help from anal physiology laboratory.

12.3 Non-relaxing Puborectalis Syndrome: Anismus

Defecation disorders occurring from functional problem rather than anatomical structure abnormalities in the anus and pelvic floor is called dyssynergic defecation, and also obstructed defecation syndrome. Here there are paradoxical puborectalis contraction, rectal hyposensitivity, and perineal descending syndrome [7, 8], we will mainly deal with paradoxical puborectalis contraction.

12.3.1 Pathophysiology

Non-relaxing puborectalis syndrome is when an abdominal pressure increases for defecation, the anal sphincter including puborectalis muscle should relax, but paradoxically, a contraction occurs, or it does not relax. These phenomena relate to excessive straining from functionally obstructed defecation in the anal canal and patients suffer from remnant due to incomplete defecation or dig out using their finger. They suffer from abdominal distension or discomfort, and in some cases accompanied with slow transit constipation. Exact cause is not defined, and it is commonly seen in women patients.

12.3.2 Examination

For the diagnosis, it is important to take detailed history taking and physical examination. In anal physiology test, electromyography and defecography are helpful and can be referred in the second chapter as it would be dealt in detail explanation (Fig. 12.1).

12.3.3 Treatment

Obstructive constipation is the same with slow transit constipation: for initial treatment, dietary therapy and medical treatment is performed. For obstructive constipation from non-relaxing puborectalis syndrome, it is not treated with surgical treatment like incision of the puborectalis muscle. The most important in constipation treatment is not the medical treatment or surgical treatment, but it is the dietary therapy starting with sufficient fiber supplement and water intake. Next step can be the proper exercise, emotional and psychological support, and correct defecation habit. Prior to the treatment, it is important to

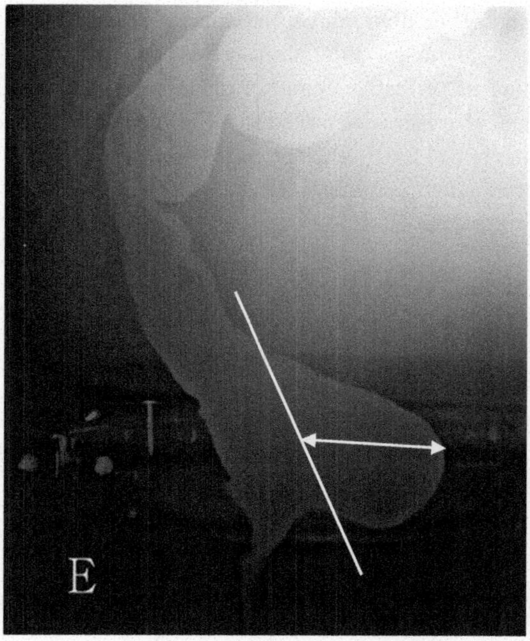

Fig. 12.1 Measurement of rectocele size: from the parallel line of the anterior rectal wall to the tip of the protrusion

confirm the patient's expectation of the treatment efficacy and degree of discomfort. As for some patients, just by understanding their defecation problem, for instance, by hearing that it is not a big disease, can make the patient deal better with the symptom and can have the patient live in a positive way [9].

12.3.3.1 Bulk-Forming Agents

In the initial treatment, it starts with dietary control and water intake then supplement with bulk-forming agents. To relieve constipation, it is recommended to take 25–30 mg of fiber a day, but as in most cases, it is not sufficient with food; therefore, additionally bulk-forming agents are administered [10]. There are also various product in sale in korea, but if it is not mixed with water properly, it is difficult to administer, and with the unpleasant taste, it is difficult to expect persistent administer from the patients. Water-soluble fiber is effective, but it tends to worsen the symptom in patient with irritable bowel syndrome suffering from gas and distention; in some cases, fiber intake should be stopped. However, it is an agent with almost no side effects, safe and effective, and generally recommended to take it prior to bedtime or before the meal, but it is best to take before breakfast right after the wake up, as for the prior to bedtime, it can make stodgy feeling.

12.3.3.2 Osmotic Agents

It is common for the patients to have taken constipation agents prior to coming to see the doctor. In osmotic agents, there are saline agents and hyperosmotic agents. The mechanism of action is that it does not absorbed in colon and increases the fluid in colon with osmotic activator [11]. The presence of sodium docuate in magnesium hydroxide can lead to hyper-magnesemia when excessive dosage is taken. In consequence, the patient with renal failure and children should be cautious. There is lactulose, sorbitol, and glycerin in hyperosmotic agents, and it can be used in the patients with difficulty in administering bulk-forming agents or with noneffective response to traditional agents. There is nonabsorbable sugar in the small intestine, fermentation by colon bacteria and change to a fatty acid which increases the osmotic action and stimulates the bowel movement. As osmotic agents do not affect blood sugar level, it can be administered in constipation patients with diabetics. They have also good efficacy in pediatrics, pregnant women, and elderly person, but one should be careful in pregnant women. Osmotic agents also decreases toxic substance formation in the bowel, removes ammonia in blood, they are used in hepatic coma. In the case with no response to these agents, stimulant agent can be used temporarily for weeks to the months. They are used as temporally purpose for short term, in the cases with long-term constipation or severe abdominal distension. The mechanism of action is, inhibit the absorption of fluid and electrolyte in the colon accumulate to promote bowel movement. But it should be cautious as osmotic agents can cause imbalance of the fluid and electrolyte, steatorrhea, protein loss, and gastroenteritis from long-term use. There are anthraquinone like aloe or senna, polyphenol like bisacodyl, and surfactant laxatives like docusate. From these, anthraquinone causes apoptosis of the epithelial cell of the large intestine and forms apoptotic body. They do phagocytosis from macrophage and form pigment-like lipofuscin, and from endoscopy it looks black, and it is called melanosis coli, and this does not look related to the structural or functional disorder of the colon [12]. Sometimes in obstructive constipation, stimulant glycerin suppository that activates only in the rectum could be effective, and if necessary, enema can be performed.

12.3.3.3 Correction in Habits and Biofeedback Treatment

Most patients with constipation have a bad habit that does not respond to normal bowel movement for defecation. For normal bowel movement, patient should be advised to go to the toilet same time every morning (in the morning or after the meal when there is gastrocolic reflex). Weight loss and exercise should be combined as it can improve bowel movement. Desire to defecate and bowel movement is a very complex and collaborated process, and part is under voluntary control, and the rest is controlled by the autonomic feedback loop. Biofeedback treatment is a method that uses many different kinds of forms and repeats this complex process for retraining. It can be performed using visual or auditory biofeedback; especially, it is a useful treatment for non-relaxing puborectalis syndrome and pelvic floor disharmony [13]. The mechanism of the treatment is structured to sense the patient's biological response and amplify, to show to the patient by converting it to a visible or auditory signal, and to train to control the targeting response. For the types, there is biofeedback using manometry or electromyography and home training unit. There is advantage in the expense as it is relatively cheap and with simple method for using electromyography rather than the manometry, and it can be done alone without equipment with only several training. For home training unit, it is usually using electromyography, and it can be trained by looking at the signal with having it connected to computer or TV. In initial biofeedback treatment, it is important to build good relationship between the patient and the therapist and should be able to advise the patients with necessary position for defecation and how to use anal and pelvic floor muscle in harmony. It is effective not only in the outlet obstructive constipation, but it is also effective in the slow transit constipation, and also it was observed to have improvement in the bowel function, decrease in dosage of defecation agent, and improvement of evaluation index in life [14–16].

12.3.3.4 Botox Injection

There are various reports on the results after improvement of symptoms in the six out of seven patients with anismus botox injection on both lateral sides of puborectalis from Hallen and others [17–19]. There is controversies on dosage of the used botox: botulinum toxin type A is commonly used, but it is generally injected on both sides of puborectalis by 10–30 units, and the author inject by 25 units. Also, patients with non-relaxing puborectalis syndrome and no efficacy with defecation agents and dietary control, then perform botox injection rather than biofeedback treatment. Negative side of botox injection is that there can be temporary gas or fecal incontinence, but in most cases, it passes away with time.

12.4 Rectocele

Rectocele is defined as anterior rectal wall and posterior vaginal wall protruding or escaping to the vagina. In some pathophysiology, extended definitions are used, including the defect of rectovaginal septum [20, 21].

12.4.1 Pathophysiology

Although the mechanism of rectocele was not clearly understood, the main cause seems to be the defect or damage of supporting fascia between the rectum and the vagina. However, fascia is not a single entity but rather a part of a more fusion form of endopelvic fascia surrounding the pelvic organs, which is directly related to their mobility and supportive function. Symptomatic rectocele is rarely seen alone and is accompanied with varying degrees of cystocele, enterocele, perineal descent, and rectal intussusceptions as a part of a broader pelvic organ support system problem. Therefore, the main risk factors of rectocele are the cause of pelvic organs prolapse. Rectocele can occur regardless of birth history, but women with birth history are considered to be the most affected group. In addition, age is related to the occurrence of rectocele, which is not a single risk factor but rather a result of complex interplay from the age-related degeneration of connective tissue, postmenopausal low-estrogen level, and the occurrence of organic disease [22].

12.4.2 Evaluation

Symptoms of the patients are mixed with various symptoms related to gynecological and bowel-related symptoms. Symptoms are constipation, obstructive defecation disorder, tenesmus, fecal incontinence, seepage, stain, pruritus, dyspareunia, pelvic pressure, and protruding lumps that can be palpated. Also, by putting hand pressure to posterior vaginal wall or perineum can facilitate bowel movement. However, symptomatic rectocele is a part of a wider range of pelvic floor dysfunction, only a minority of these symptoms is directly related to rectocele.

Examination can be done having the patient in left lateral decubitus and strain to confirm the protrusion of the posterior vaginal wall or can observe perineal descent. Also, by defecography, the size of rectocele can be measured. Having parallel line on the anterior rectal wall as a baseline, the degree of protrusion over the baseline is the size of rectum (Fig. 12.1) [23]. MRI defecography or dynamic perineal ultrasound is also used [24].

12.4.3 Treatment

12.4.3.1 Medical Treatment

Although rectocele suffering from outlet obstructive constipation symptom can be improved by medical treatment together with lifestyle change, in the case with weak response, surgery has to be considered. Medical treatments, like general constipation treatments, should have the patient administer fiber, drink plenty of water, if necessary, increase laxatives. There is controversy about the efficacy of biofeedback therapy, but if there is levator ani syndrome accompanied, it can be attempted prior to the surgery. In addition, considerable number of patients with outlet obstructive constipation can have psychiatric problem accompanied, if necessary, psychiatric treatment should be performed prior to the surgery.

12.4.3.2 Surgical Treatment

Prior to the surgical treatment, sufficient examination should be performed to determine whether there are any other outlet obstructive causes, and surgery has to be considered only when there is no response to non-operative treatment. Also, there should be sufficient consultation on the possibility of continuing of postoperative medical treatment, or even after the surgery, there could still be outlet obstructive constipation [25]. There are various methods in surgical treatment, and the comparison of results is not easy, due to difficulty in follow-up examination and patient's symptoms and measurement methods.

Even after a generally used surgery, the change in the size of rectocele is not significantly correlated with the improvement of symptom. Surgical method is to reinforce the posterior vaginal wall or strengthen the anterior rectal wall. Another method is to reinforce the graft or tissue interposition between the rectum and the posterior vaginal wall. Recently, it is reported of abdominal approach using laparoscope, and using auto-stapler the incised anterior rectal wall and strengthening the anterior wall to reduce the rectal redundancy method (STARR) [26].

Transvaginal Repair (Posterior Colporrhaphy)

Some of the colorectal surgeons and most of the gynecologists prefer this surgical method. The surgery is performed in lithotomy position under spinal anesthesia, and a transverse incision is made at the cross point of the mucosa of vagina entrance and perineum, and then a vertical incision is made toward the vaginal apex. Dissect delicately the posterior vaginal wall from the underlying fibromuscular layer. Vaginal wall is dissected up to rectocele and laterally, to the medical edge of the puborectalis. A midline plication of fibromuscular tissue and the levator muscles is performed in an interrupted fashion using an absorbable suture (3–0 vicryl). Redundant vaginal mucosa is excised and sutured in the same way to normalize the vaginal hiatus. Other than plication of the levator muscle and fibromuscular layer, surgical procedure is same as the traditional posterior colporrhaphy (Fig. 12.2).

The success of the surgery depends largely on the experience of the surgeon, starting with identifying the accurate defect range of rectocele, and during the surgery, measuring it with the inserted index finger in the anus. Rectovaginal septum is composed mainly of thin endopelvic fascia and is weakened by the break of normal fascia attached to perineum. It is very important to reinforce the septum during the surgery. As prosthesis or biologic graft is additionally inserted, it is considered to be reinforced theoretically; however, there was no significant difference from the study [27, 28].

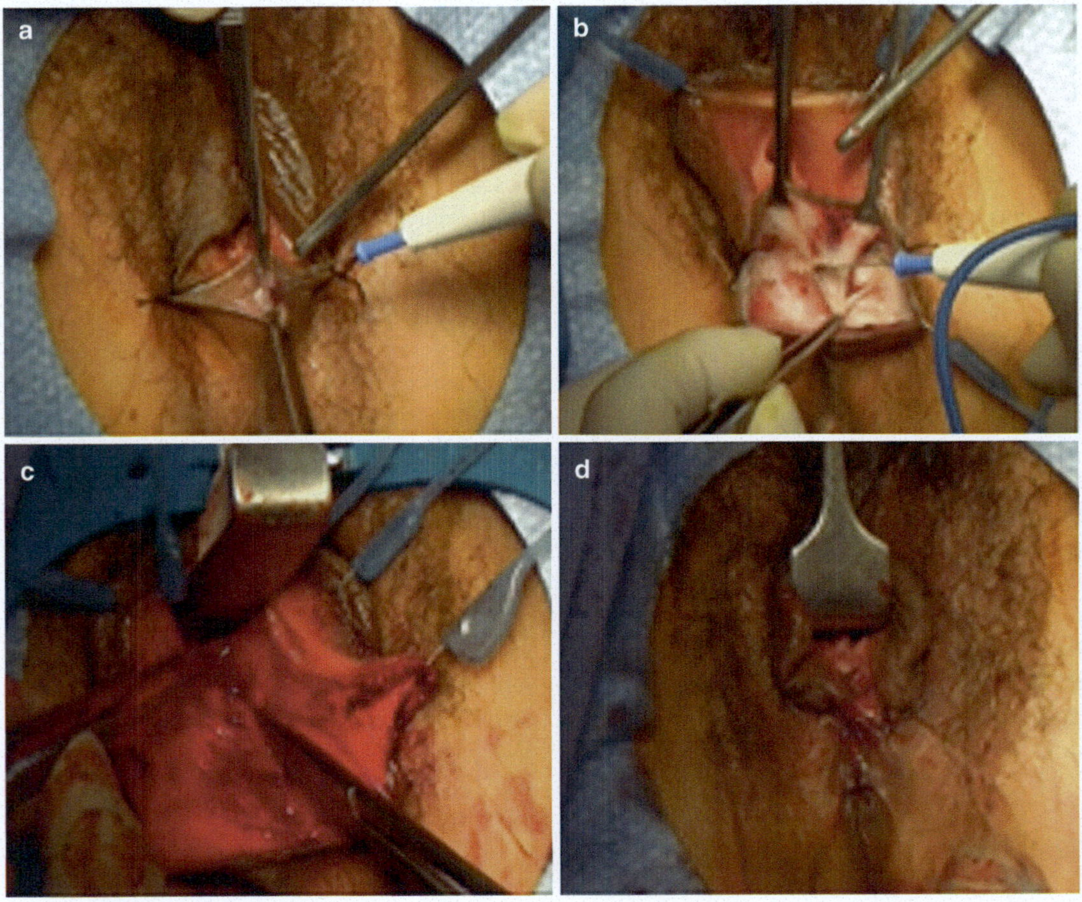

Fig. 12.2 Transperineal or transvaginal approach for the rectocele. (**a**) In lithotomy position, a transverse incision is made at the perineum. (**b**) Posterior vaginal wall is dissected from the underlying fibromuscular layer. (**c**) The fibromuscular tissue and levator muscles is sutured. (**d**) The perineum was repaired by vertical interrupted suture

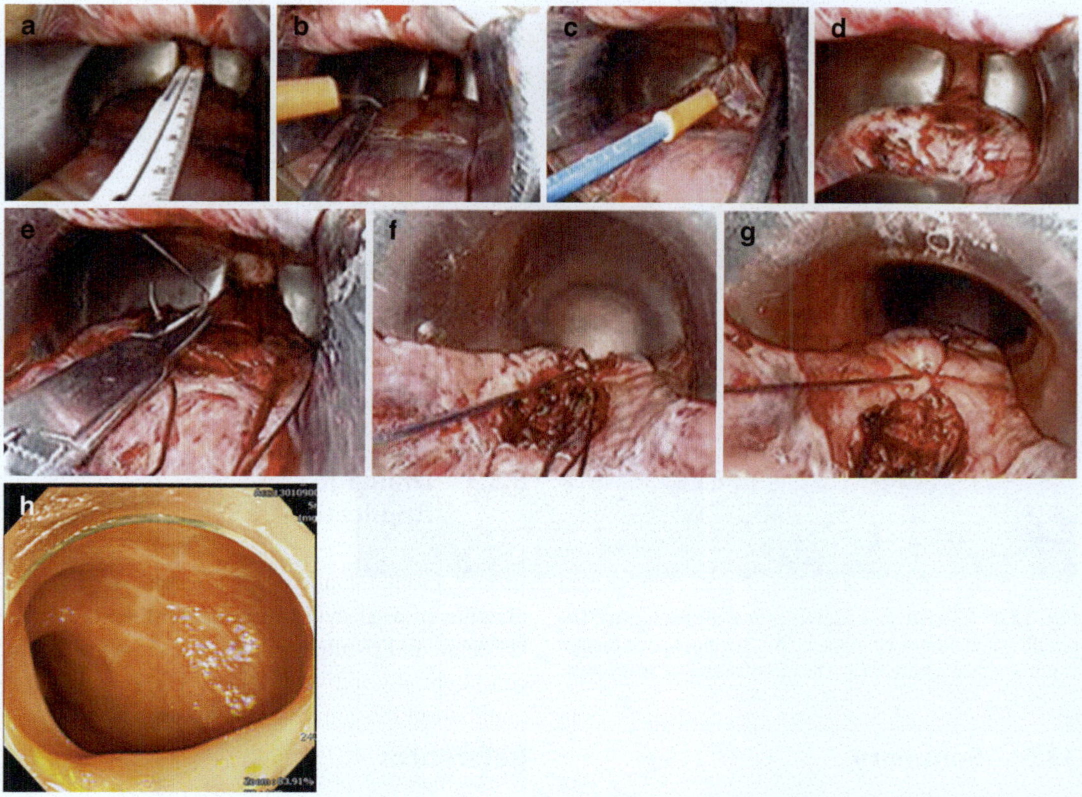

Fig. 12.3 Transanal approach for the rectocele. (**a**) In jackknife position, bivalved retractor is applied. (**b**) A transverse incision is made from dentate line. (**c**) Then, vertical incision is made like inverted T-shape. (**d**) Fully dissection is made along the submucosal layer. (**e**) Rectal muscular layer is sutured. (**f**) Plication with interrupted absorbable sutures transversely or longitudinally. (**g**) Rectal mucosal layer is sutured. (**h**) Endoscopic findings of sutured wound after healing

Transanal Repair

With long-term rectocele, the anterior rectal wall becomes thin and mucosa stretches. Transanal surgery is to strengthen the thinned rectal wall and excise the extra mucosa [29]. Surgery is performed in prone jack knife position with a bivalved retractor, and epinephrine-mixed saline is injected into submucosal layer to reduce intraoperative bleeding and facilitate dissection. It is fully dissected along the submucosal layer with inverted T-shaped incision from the dentate line and dissected together with extra mucosa. Rectal muscular layer is plicated with interrupted absorbable sutures transversely or longitudinally. Be cautious not to suture together the vaginal wall as it can cause postoperative recto-vaginal fistula (Fig. 12.3). The recurrence rate is known to be higher than the transvaginal approach; however, the surgery is relatively simple, and as there are almost no postoperative complications like dyspareunia, it is a recommended method in young women [30–32].

There's also rectocele surgery using auto-stapler device, with less bleeding and short surgery time, and initially it was used, but with reports of several severe complications and high incidence of recurrence from long-term follow-up tests, now it is no longer commonly used [33–36].

STARR (Stapled Transanal Resection of the Rectum) (Fig. 12.4)

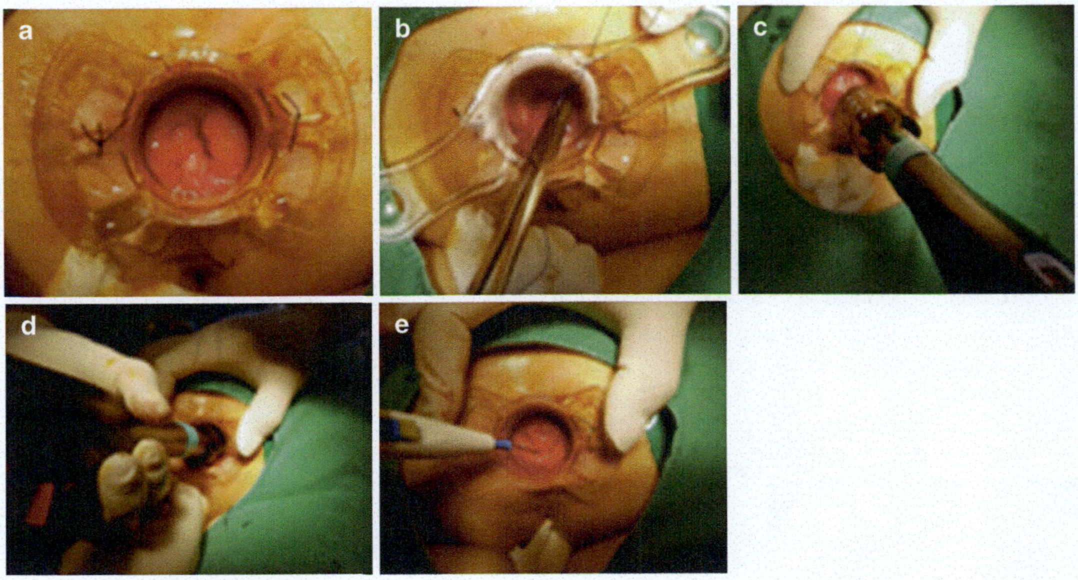

Fig. 12.4 STARR procedure for the rectocele. (**a**) The circular anal dilator is applied. (**b**) The mucosa of rectum is purse string sutured. (**c**) The circular stapler is inserted. (**d**) After closing, circular stapler is fired. (**e**) Check the bleeding and intact anastomosis

12.5 Summary

It is not easy to choose an appropriate surgical method as the lack of prospective studies in rectocele surgery, differences in selection of surgical patient, and evaluation on postoperative results varies. There was no difference in postoperative recurrence and no comparison in functional outcome from comparative study of the transanal or transvaginal repair. Rectocele is a functional disease with structural problems; through detailed medical history and physical examination and anal physiology tests, accompanied pelvic floor diseases should be examined. Prior to the surgery, change in lifestyle, if necessary, psychiatric treatment, and surgery should be considered for the patients with no response to the medical treatment for at least over 6 months. The surgery is relatively simple, effective, and safe method and shows good results with short-term follow-up, but as the clinical outcome of long-term follow-up is controversial, it should be discussed with the patient prior to the surgery.

References

1. Gordon PH. Anorectal anatomy and physiology. Gastroenterol Clin N Am. 2001;30:1–13.
2. Palit S, Lunniss PJ, Scott SM. The physiology of human defecation. Dig Dis Sci. 2012;57(6):1445–64.
3. Bajwa A, Thiruppathy K, Trivedi P, Boulos P, Emmanuel A. Effect of rectal distension on voluntary external anal sphincter function in healthy subjects. Color Dis. 2011;13(10):1173–9.
4. Brookes SJ, Dinning PG, Gladman MA. Neuroanatomy and physiology of colorectal function and defaecation: from basic science to human clinical studies. Neurogastroenterol Motil. 2009;21 Suppl 2:9–19.
5. Bharucha AE, Rao SS. An update on anorectal disorders for gastroenterologists. Gastroenterology. 2014;146(1):37–45.
6. Rao SS, Welcher KD, Leistikow JS. Obstructive defecation: a failure of rectoanal coordination. Am J Gastroenterol. 1998;93(7):1042–50.
7. Andromanakos N, Skandalakis P, Troupis T, Filippou D. Constipation of anorectal outlet obstruction: pathophysiology, evaluation and management. J Gastroenterol Hepatol. 2006;21(4):638–46.
8. Higgins PD, Johanson JF. Epidemiology of constipation in North America: a systematic review. Am J Gastroenterol. 2004;99(4):750–9.

9. Podzemny V, Pescatori LC, Pescatori M. Management of obstructed defecation. World J Gastroenterol. 2015;21(4):1053–60.
10. Pucciani F, Raggioli M, Ringressi MN. Usefulness of psyllium in rehabilitation of obstructed defecation. Tech Coloproctol. 2011;15(4):377–83.
11. Bharucha AE. Difficult defecation: difficult problem assessment and management; what really helps? Gastroenterol Clin N Am. 2011;40(4):837–44.
12. Chatoor D, Emmnauel A. Constipation abd evacuation disorders. Best Pract Res Clin Gastroenterol. 2009;23:517–30.
13. Rao SS, Welcher KD, Pelsang RE. Effects of biofeedback therapy on anorectal function in obstructive defecation. Dig Dis Sci. 1997;42(11):2197–205.
14. Heyman S, Scarlett Y, Jones K, Ringel Y, Drossman D, et al. Randomized, controlled trial shows biofeedback to be superior to alternative treatments for patients with pelvic floor dyssnyneria-type constipation. Dis Colon Rectum. 2007;50:428–41.
15. Chiotakakou-Faliakou E, Kamm MA, Roy AJ, Storrie JP, Turner IC. Biofeedback provides long-term benefit for patients with intractable, slow and normal transit constipation. Gut. 1998;42:517–21.
16. Brown SR, Donti D, Seow-Choen F, Ho YH. Biofeedback avoids surgery in patients with slow-transit constipation: report of four cases. Dis Colon Rectum. 2001;44:737–9.
17. Hallan RI, Williams NS, Melling J, Waldron DJ, Womack NR, Morrison JFB. Treatment of anismus in intractable constipation with botulinum. Lancet. 1988;2:714–7.
18. Joo JS, Agachan F, Wolff B, Nogueras JJ, Wexner SD. Initial north American experience with botulinum toxin type a for treatment of anismus. Dis Colon Rectum. 1996;39:1107–11.
19. Ron Y, Avni Y, Lukovetski A, et al. Botulinum toxin type a in therapy of patients with anismus. Dis Colon Rectum. 2001;44:1821–6.
20. Guzman Rojas R, Quintero C, Shek KL, Dietz HP. Does childbirth play a role in the etiology of rectocele? Int Urogynecol J. May 2015;26(5):737–41.
21. Mellgren A, Bremmer S, Johansson C, et al. Defecography. Results of investigations in 2,816 patients. Dis Colon Rectum. Nov. 1994;37(11):1133–41.
22. Mustain WC. Functional disorders: rectocele. Clin Colon Rectal Surg. 2017;30(1):63–75.
23. Hicks CW1, Weinstein M, Wakamatsu M, Pulliam S, Savitt L, Bordeianou L. Are rectoceles the cause or the result of obstructed defaecation syndrome? A prospective anorectal physiology study. Color Dis 2013;15(8):993–999.
24. Puigdollers A, Fernández-Fraga X, Azpiroz F. Persistent symptoms of functional outlet obstruction after rectocele repair. Color Dis. 2007;9(3):262–5.
25. Piloni V, Tosi P, Vernelli M. MR-defecography in obstructed defecation syndrome (ODS): technique, diagnostic criteria and grading. Tech Coloproctol. 2013;17(5):501–10.
26. Paraiso MF, Barber MD, Muir TW, Walters MD. Rectocele repair: a randomized trial of three surgical techniques including graft augmentation. Am J Obstet Gynecol. 2006;195(6):1762–71.
27. Abramov Y, Gandhi S, Goldberg RP, Botros SM, Kwon C, Sand PK. Site-specific rectocele repair compared with standard posterior colporrhaphy. Obstet Gynecol. 2005;105(2):314–8.
28. Porter WE, Steele A, Walsh P, Kohli N, Karram MM. The anatomic and functional outcomes of defect-specific rectocele repairs. Am J Obstet Gynecol. 1999;181(6):1353–8.
29. Fabiani P, Benizri E, Gugenheim J, Mouiel J. Surgical treatment of anterior rectoceles in women. The transanal approach. Ann Chir. 2000;125(8):779–81.
30. Marks MM. The rectal side of the rectocele. Dis Colon Rectum. 1967;10:387–8.
31. Nieminen K, Hiltunen KM, Laitinen J, Oksala J, Heinonen PK. Transanal or vaginal approach to rectocele repair: a prospective, randomized pilot study. Dis Colon Rectum. 2004;47(10):1636–42.
32. Roman H, Michot F. Long-term outcomes of transanal rectocele repair. Dis Colon Rectum. 2005;48(3):510–7.
33. Harris MA, Ferrara A, Gallagher J, DeJesus S, Williamson P, Larach S. Stapled transanal rectal resection vs. transvaginal rectocele repair for treatment of obstructive defecation syndrome. Dis Colon Rectum. 2009;52(4):592–7.
34. Pescatori M, Dodi G, Salafia C, Zbar AP. Rectovaginal fistula after double-stapled transanal rectotomy (STARR) for obstructed defaecation. Int J Color Dis. 2005;20:83–5.
35. Asteria CR, Bellarosa S, Chiarioni G, Mazzola F, Bruni O, Villanacci V, Bassotti G. Long-term follow-up of after STARR for obstructed defecation. Tech Coloproctol. 2014;18:213–4.
36. Mahmoud SA, Omar W, Farid M. Transanal repair for treatment of rectocele in obstructed defaecation: manual or stapled. Color Dis. 2012;14(1):104–10.

13 Fecal Incontinence

Jung Ryul Oh

13.1 Introduction

Fecal incontinence generally refers to a condition of sudden stool leak from the anus repeatedly without control for over 1 month and in the age above 5 years. The incidence of incontinence increases in elderly and the quality of life deteriorates. Anal continence is controlled by complex interaction of pelvic floor muscle, anal sphincter, rectal compliance, stool consistency, and cognitive function. The cause of incontinence can vary and can be classified as primary incontinence (congenital malformation) or secondary incontinence (acquired conditions). Primary incontinence (congenital malformation) is most commonly seen in infant or child incontinence caused by meningitis, Hirschsprung's disease, anorectal atresia, and anorectal anomaly surgery. Neurological causes can also be caused by abnormalities of cerebral palsy, upper or lower neurological disease, and internal pudendal nerve which controls the anal sphincter. The main causes of secondary incontinence are birth injury and anal surgery (hemorrhoid, fistula, and fissure). In anal sonography, anal sphincter damage can be found from 35% of women with vaginal delivery. In addition, pudendal nerve injury due to pregnancy and childbirth is an invisible damage, but it can be the cause of incontinence. The cause of incontinence is quite diverse, and it is generally known to occur with various complex factors; therefore, patient's history should be taken in detail [1, 2].

13.2 Diagnostic Evaluation

13.2.1 History Taking

In patients with incontinence, it is essential to ask about the patient's past history in detail. Patients with fecal incontinence tend to be uncomfortable in talking about their symptoms, so detail questioning should be done during examination. Uncontrolled stool or gas leakage is associated with decreased sensation, anorectal reflex dysfunction, or abnormal function of anal sphincter muscle. When trying to tolerate defecation, but the stool or gas is leaking, this indicates dysfunction of anal sphincter muscle or decrease in the rectal compliance. When the stool is leaked after defecation, it can occur with incomplete defecation or deteriorated rectal sensation. Having patients write a daily diary of their symptoms can help determining the direction of examination and treatment, and also it can be useful in determining the efficacy of the treatment. In addition to the identification of underlying disease, the cause of disease can be analogized by questioning during examination, number and time of defecation, number and time of incontinence, stool consistency, number

J. R. Oh (✉)
Colorectal Division, Department of Surgery, Hansol Hospital, Seoul, South Korea

D. K. Lee (ed.), *Practices of Anorectal Surgery*, https://doi.org/10.1007/978-981-13-1447-6_13

and time of rectal urgency, and use of pads and drugs [3].

13.2.2 Physical Examination

In physical examination, digital rectal examination including the perineum is the basic examination. By observing the presence of stool around the anus, protruding hemorrhoids, dermatitis or scar around the anus, or whether the anus is open will determine the dysfunction of the sphincter muscle or chronic skin irritation. When perianal skin is tapped lightly with cotton swab, in normal cases, contraction of the external sphincter occurs, but if the anodermal reflex has disappeared, this indicates the damage of afferent or efferent innervation. Through digital rectal examination, you can examine the resting pressure of the anal canal, degree of squeezing pressure, pressure change of the sphincter muscle in defecation, and degree of perineal descent [4].

13.2.3 Endoscopic and Radiologic Examination

Endoscopy is appropriate for detecting mucosal lesion or tumor or the rectum, and anal ultrasonography is useful for identifying structural defects of the anal sphincter muscle and condition of the puborectalis muscle. Anal ultrasonography is especially useful for detecting the structural defects of anal sphincter muscle and for checking the thickness of internal and external sphincter muscle [5]. Magnetic resonance imaging is known to be a good method to identify external sphincter, the rectum, or structure around the rectum [6]. Defecography is used to diagnose anorectal angle, pelvic descent, and rectal prolapse, but it is a limited examination for diagnosing fecal incontinence [7].

13.2.4 Anorectal Physiologic Testing

Anorectal manometry and rectal sensory tests are good tools to determine the abnormalities of the internal and external sphincter function and sensory of the rectum. Anorectal manometry measures resting and squeezing pressure of the anal sphincter muscle, pressure of compression, rectal sensory, anorectal reflex, and rectal compliance [8]. Patients with fecal incontinence show lower sphincter pressure or decrease in rectal sensory. Balloon expulsion test is a simple test that can be used to determine the dysfunction of defecation in the patients with leaking stool after defecation or in the patients with fecal impaction or obstructive defecation.

13.2.5 Assessment of Severity and Impact on Quality of Life

Grading of the severity of fecal incontinence is an objective tool for assessing the response of before and after treatment and comparing the data from each hospital. The most widely used assessment tools are the Cleveland Clinic Florida Fecal Incontinence Score (CCF-FI), Fecal Incontinence Severity Index (FISI), and Fecal Incontinence Quality of Life Scale (FIQL).

13.3 Treatment

13.3.1 Non-operative Treatment

13.3.1.1 Supportive Treatment

In supportive treatment, the patient should avoid food or activity that can cause symptom and try to have regular bowel habit, and it is important to pay attention to perianal skin hygiene, reduce intake of caffeine and fiber, and restrain postprandial activity to minimize irregular defecation.

13.3.1.2 Medical Treatment

The purpose of medication is to reduce the number of defecation or to improve the consistency of stool. By using antidiarrheal agent like loperamide or diphenoxylate/atropine, it can reduce the number of defecations [9, 10]. Initially, loperamide can be taken starting with 2–4 mg/day increasing up to 16 mg/day; it can improve the rectal elasticity by reducing urgency and strengthening the internal sphincter muscle. However, it needs caution, as it can have side effects like abdominal distension or pain, constipation, nausea, vomiting, and fecal impaction [10]. In unknown causes of fecal incontinence, the efficacy of amitriptyline from antidepressant agent was identified from limited studies. By administering 20 mg every night before bedtime for 4 weeks, it was reported to show improvement in the incontinence symptoms. The mechanism of action is presumed to be that the anticholinergic action of amitriptyline slows decreasing the rectal motility [11].

13.3.1.3 Biofeedback Therapy

Biofeedback therapy is a noninvasive treatment that strengthens the pelvic floor muscles and abdominal wall muscles through cognitive training. Repetitive training can increase strength of the anal sphincter and improve compression of voluntary anal sphincter after feeling the sense in the rectum and can increase the anorectal sensory [12–14]. Training anal sphincter to have voluntary maximal compression within 2 seconds after the dilatation of inserted balloon from the rectum. However, efficacy of biofeedback therapy is low if accompanied by the following abnormalities like severe fecal incontinence, pudendal nerve dysfunction, and nervous system abnormalities [15, 16]. Although there are differences in the results of each studies, because the method is not standardized, many studies on biofeedback therapy show its efficacy in fecal incontinence treatment; therefore, it is recommended to patients with difficulties in improving symptoms from supportive treatment alone [4].

13.3.1.4 Bulking Agent Injection

Fifteen percent to twenty percent of resting anal pressure is maintained from the hemorrhoidal plexus, rare, but suffers from passive incontinence after hemorrhoid surgery, internal sphincterotomy on anal fissure, or simple fistulotomy. For bulking agent, there are Solesta®, Permacol®, Durasphere®, and from those, FDA-approved Solesta® is used [17–20]. We have experience in using Permacol®, it was simple to use, and the short-term result was outstanding. Durasphere® was mainly used for urinary incontinence and then introduced to the fecal incontinence.

The treatment can be performed in the surgery room without anesthesia. Enema and injection of prophylactic antibiotics is performed prior to the surgery. The needle should reach submucosal layer above the dentate line from the anus through the intersphincteric space (Fig. 13.1). The injection dosage is 2–3 ml, and it does not need to be done under anal ultrasonography as swelling can be identified visually. Direct injection to the mucosa should be avoided due to leakage of bulking agent. In some cases, it is injected in the intersphincteric space, but it should be injected in the submucosal layer above the dentate line.

13.3.1.5 Radio-Frequency Energy Delivery

Using specialized energy delivery system, anoscopy (SECCA), incontinence is treated by increasing the thickness of propria muscle layer with structural change of collagen cell from firing the radio-frequency energy to the internal sphincter in the inner side of the anal mucosa [21–23]. The anoscopy of this system has on one side bent injection needles aligned in 5 mm interval with nickel titanium. It brings up the internal sphincter temperature up to 85° by firing the radio-frequency energy from the lower anal canal moving to the upper anal canal. At this time, have cold water running to avoid increase of temperature in the mucosa layer. The treatment can be performed in the surgery room under intravenous anesthesia in prone jackknife position. It is performed at the lower and upper dentate line about 4–5 levels in 4 directions, and one should be cautious not to insert needle too deep in the anterior side of the anus in women patients.

13.3.2 Operative Treatment

Operative treatment can be considered after the safe and simple methods like supportive therapy, medication treatment, and biofeedback therapy have failed. The most commonly used surgical methods are sphincteroplasty to restore the anal sphincter and pelvic floor muscles and other neuromodulatory procedures that augment the anal sphincter. If the procedure is inappropriate or unsuccessful, enterostomy can be chosen as the next treatment, but it is not preferred in most patients. In particular, it is known to be an appropriate treatment for the patients with spinal cord injury and paralysis patients associated with complications due to incontinence [24]. In this chapter, we will mainly focus on the sphincter restoration surgery for incontinence after birth injury.

13.3.2.1 Sphincteroplasty

Surgery of sphincter rupture by injury originates from the overlapping sphincteroplasty described by Parks [19], (Fig. 13.2). Sphincteroplasty is used in

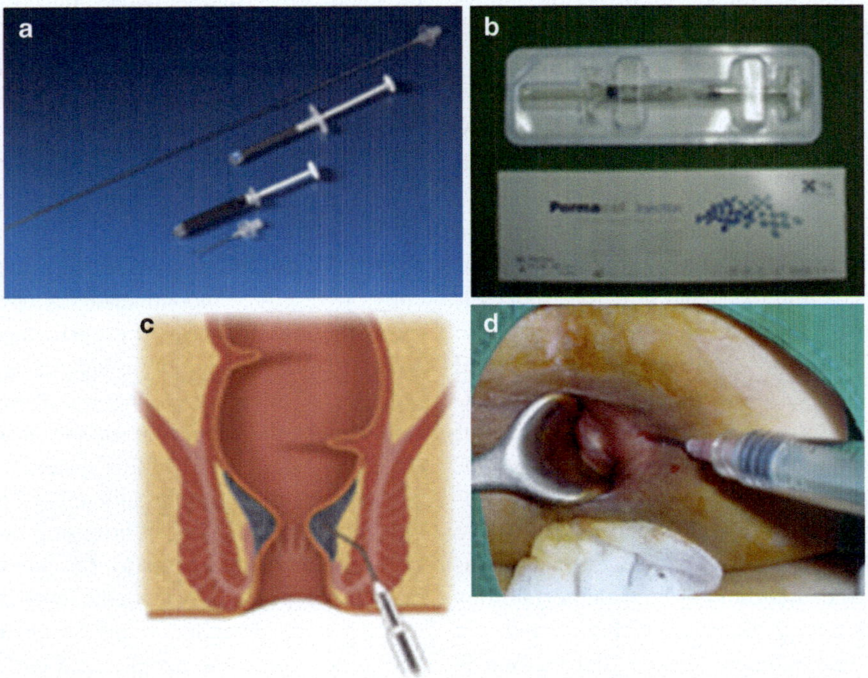

Fig. 13.1 Bulking agent injection (**a**) Injectable bulking agents with syringe. (**b**) Permacol® is simple to use. (**c**, **d**) Submucosal injection of bulking agent around internal anal sphincter

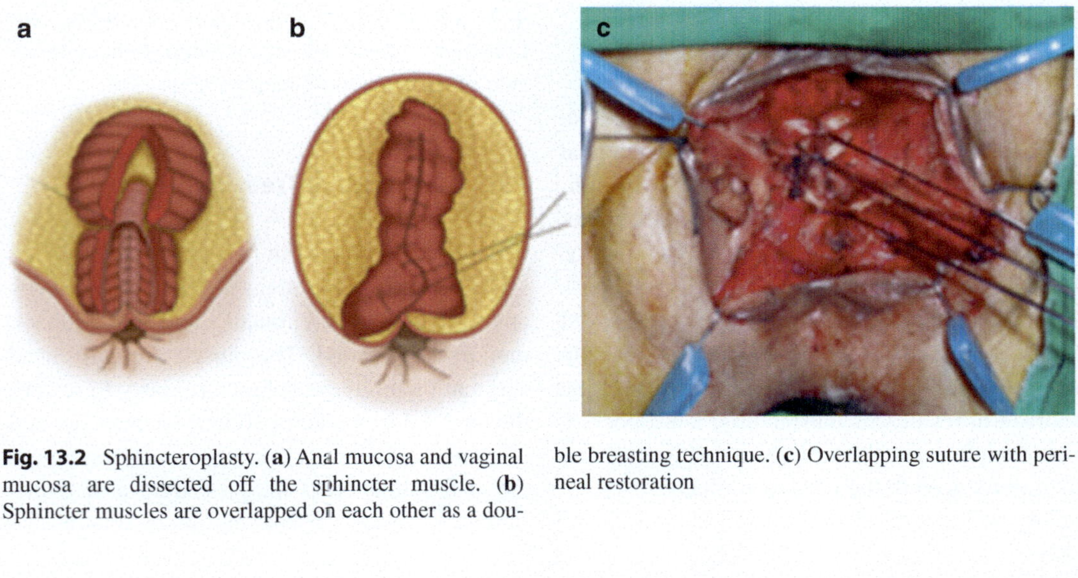

Fig. 13.2 Sphincteroplasty. (**a**) Anal mucosa and vaginal mucosa are dissected off the sphincter muscle. (**b**) Sphincter muscles are overlapped on each other as a double breasting technique. (**c**) Overlapping suture with perineal restoration

patients with visible damage of the external sphincter muscle, and most of them have gone through anal fistula surgery or have obstetrical injury. This method is less successful if the extent of damaged sphincter is too wide or too old, and the faster the surgery, the better the result [25–27]. In general, in the case surgery wound is not infected and there is no evidence of neurogenic fecal incontinence, the results are good. Therefore, it is considered to be the best treatment in the case with partial or complete rupture of the external sphincter. In the case with sphincter rupture due to birth injury, it may need perineal restoration surgery due to the cloacogenic deformity by complete separation of the sphincter muscle. In the case of failed surgery after immediate repair following birth injury, the surgery has to wait at least 6 months for the surrounding tissue to be stabilized. Surgery is performed under spinal anesthesia in lithotomy position.

Stage 1

Use Lone Star Retractor; place it in the anus, perineum, and vaginal orifice to secure surgical view. Inject epinephrine-mixed saline along the incision site to prevent bleeding. Transverse curvilinear incision is made along the perineal region between the anus and the vagina, but it must not go beyond the medial half of the anus to prevent damage in the branch of the pudendal nerve. Through delicate dissection from the vaginal wall and the anal mucosa, identify the tear in the sphincter and fully dissect from the surrounding subcutaneous fat tissue without separating the internal and the external sphincter. After scar tissue is cut, dissect laterally along the healthy muscle allowing the cut muscles to overlap with at least 1.5 cm margin. If necessary, dissect between the rectum and the vagina and have bulbospongiosus muscle confirmed.

Stage 2

Clean the wound area thoroughly and slightly loosen the retractor. Then, simple interrupt suture anal mucosa to the anal verge using the 3-0 Vicryl. Overlapping suture is done with pulling the separated muscle to the center; at this time, mattress suture is performed using 3-0 Prolene, nonabsorbable suture, and be cautious not to suture too tight, as it can cause ischemic change. In the case with difficulty in overlapping suture, end-to-end anastomosis of the sphincter muscle can be performed, but there should be no tension after the suture. In cloacogenic deformity, restore pelvic floor muscles by simple interrupted suture of the bulbospongiosus muscle with a slight pull.

Stage 3

After suturing the muscle layer, the skin suturing should be done in a longitudinal suture on lateral incision to have an elongated effect on anal canal and perineum which increases the anal function and form new perineal body. Insert drain tube if dead space is likely to appear when suturing, but it is important to prevent accumulation of discharge and bleeding, by suturing sufficiently on not only the sphincter but also the soft tissue. Then, clean the wound and place suction drain if the dead space is determined to be big, and insert Foley catheter (Fig. 13.3).

Prior to the sphincteroplasty, we performed bowel preparation according to the colonoscopy, and immediately before surgery, prophylactic antibiotics the second-generation cephalosporin and metronidazole are injected intravenously. After the operation, the same antibiotic is injected intravenously for about 2–3 days, and then, oral antibiotic is administered for 3–5 days. The inserted Foley catheter is maintained for 3–5 days, and defecation is restrained by using antidiarrhea agent, and the wound is daily dressed. After, warm sitz bath should be done 3–4 times a day and administer stool softener and bulking agent, and it is important to train the patient not to be strain during defecation. Patients with satisfactory result gain ability to control bowel movement after 6–8 weeks. Patients are recommended to do pelvic rehabilitation exercise after the operation, which is considered to improve the function.

It is important to have enough sphincters in overlapping sphincteroplasty, but as it can cause ischemia and damage pudendal nerve, if the dissection is performed more than the degree, it is better to avoid dissecting over 3 or 9 o'clock from the sphincteroplasty. In the case with sphincter muscle injuries and despite the corrective surgery, if the symptoms persist, this is because in most cases, there will be persistent sphincter injury. In this case, it could be that there

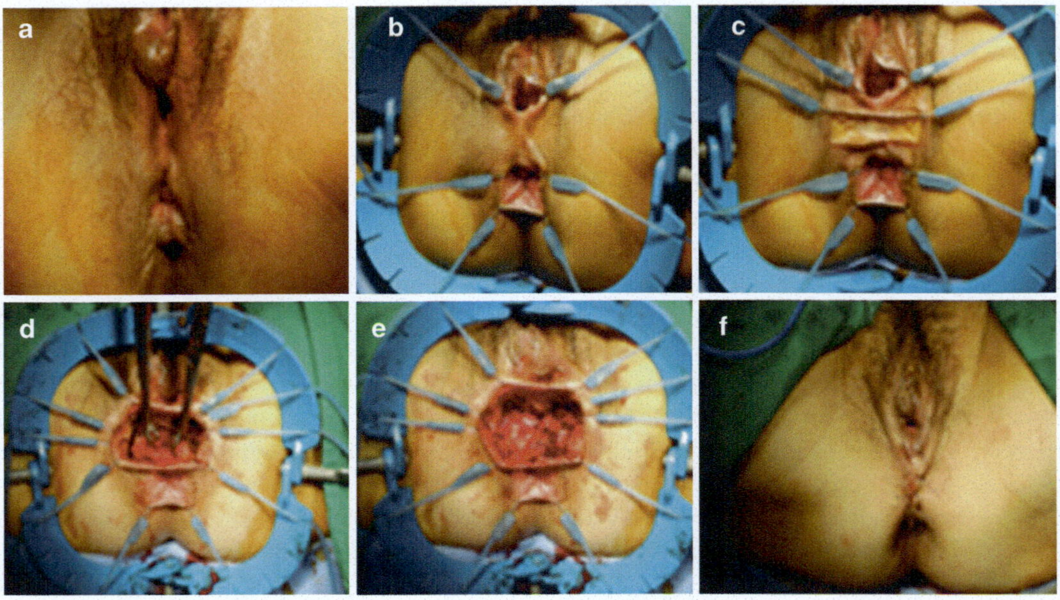

Fig. 13.3 Triple plasty for cloacogenic deformity including sphincteroplasty, levatoplasty, and perineoplasty. (**a**) Preoperatively, cloacogenic deformity. (**b**) Lone Star Retractor is used and placed in the anus, perineum, and vaginal orifice. (**c**) Transverse curvilinear incision is made along the perineal region between the anus and the vagina. (**d**) Delicate dissection from vaginal wall and anal mucosa with sufficient dissection laterally along the healthy muscle. (**e**) Overlapping suture with pulling the separated muscle to the center. (**f**) After operation, form new perineal body

was insufficient sphincteroplasty during the operation or the operation was done sufficiently, but the surgical region was not maintained well due to scar tissue or muscle hypotrophy in the elderly.

Insufficient dissection in the overlapping sphincteroplasty can be the cause of postoperative recurrence as it can create too much tension in the suture area. And if insufficient sphincteroplasty is determined and revision is performed on the same site, it can increase the possibility of sphincter control nerve damage or cause ischemia or scarring on the surrounding tissue; therefore revision should be performed up to two times and no more than three times. Revision should be performed on the basis of determining that persistent damage from ultrasonography and that the function of the external sphincter are at least maintained like the initial operation [28–31].

13.3.2.2 Posterior Repair

Posterior repair is performed in the patients with idiopathic or neurogenic incontinence and with mild external sphincter injury. It is similar to the plication method in sphincteroplasty, but the difference is that the range is broader and fundamentally, the plication is performed on the pelvic floor muscles. It can be considered as a plication process for the levator muscle, and sphincter plication is in most cases included in the process. The principle of the operation is to go through intersphincteric plane to expose pubococcygeus, puborectalis, and iliococcygeal muscles and suture the posterior part of these muscles and also suture posterior part of external sphincter.

The operation is performed in jackknife position with round incision along the anal verge in the posterior half and dissect subcutaneous tissue placing at least 4 cm away from posterior side of the anus. The skin flap is thickened until the posterior fibers of external sphincter muscle are visible. Identify medial fibers of the external sphincter and pull it backward. The next step in the operation is to dissect intersphincteric plane. With deeper dissection, pull the rectum forward using small retractor. Afterward, as the rectum is pulled forward, cut Waldeyer's fascia laterally. An incomplete cut of Waldeyer's fascia will lead to inadequate separation of the rectum from the sacrum which will cause insufficient exposure of the levator muscle. If there is insufficient space between the muscles on the both sides of the puborectalis muscle, it is difficult to perform proper repair surgery. Repair is done with two layers or one-layer suture. In the case of layer by layer suture, suture the puborectalis muscle first, and then suture iliococcygeus and pubococcygeus muscle as second layer. Second layer suturing is to reinforce the prior sutured layer.

Kipley and others have reported that in the posterior repair, there was no postoperative complication other than extensive bruising and small skin necrosis. Out of 124 patients, extensive bruising occurred in 21% and skin necrosis occurred in 25%. Bruise is considered to be a hematoma formed after the operation with disappearance of weak adrenaline solution effect. Therefore, in the case with an insufficient hemostasis rather than using adrenaline, suction drainage is installed. And the wound infection occurred only in 11%. Twelve of these patients had rectal injury, but only two cases had fistula, and both cases were successfully healed with mucosa advancement flap.

13.3.2.3 Sacral Nerve Stimulation

Fundamentally sacral nerve stimulation (SNS) is applied to fecal incontinence due to damage or degenerative changes of internal sphincter muscle and due to weakening of tension from other reasons although the external sphincter is structurally normal. It is presumed that the fecal incontinence is improved with inserted electrodes in the S3 bony hole which stimulates with low intensity to improve the function of the rectum, sensory, and anal sphincter muscle [32–34]. Three years of follow-up in the prospective, multicenter studies showed that 86% of the patients had more than 50% reduction in the incidence of incontinence and a significantly lower incidence of incontinence per week compared to the prior to the procedure [35]. In the early days, it was mainly used in the patients with no structural defects or with less anal sphincter muscle injury, but recently, it is reported to be effective in the patients with defects in anal sphincter muscle [36]. It is a relatively old treatment method, but recently the function and the methods have been developed, and now neurostimulator can be inserted under local anesthesia in the outpatients and can be switched on and off and controlled by a remote control [37]. Prior to the permanent insertion of the device, it can have a test period, which enables to confirm the effectiveness, and it has advantage of being relatively safe procedure and low in complications compared to the other surgical treatment. There is also extracorporeal magnetic stimulation (EMS) derived from the SNS. When stimulated with magnetic field, it creates electric field that can cause polarization of nerve membrane, and for this, magnetic field is used to stimulate as a noninvasive means in the sacral nerve in vitro. However, since this method is influenced by the body shape of the patient which makes it difficult to expect a sufficient effect, recently, a method of direct stimulation to pudendal nerve by applying magnetic field directly on the perineum is also used. Stimulating pudendal nerve and stimulating sacral nerve, their backgrounds are theoretically different. However, considering the principle of biofeedback therapy, EMS can be expected to have a significant effect in that the stimulation of pudendal nerve, whether it is caused by a magnetic field or not, should also be effective [38–40].

Some patients do not have incontinence improvement despite the repeated surgical efforts, and eventually they need to create an enterostomy. Many of these patients feel relieved that to some degree, it is possible for them to have control over defecation despite the inconvenience of having to carry the device. In some patients with severely aggravated anal function, enterostomy is recommended in the first meeting; however, most of the patients accept ostomy only after all other efforts have failed.

13.4 Summary

There are various causes and degrees in a fecal incontinence. A number of treatment methods are attempted, but still there's lack of standard guideline on which treatment should be used in which cases. It is desirable to take a comprehensive consideration prior to choosing a method, the cause of incontinence, accompanied disease, general condition, risk and contraindication of procedure, and mechanism of the treatment and should take staged approach examining response to the treatment. There is still lack of effective treatment for severe fecal incontinence; more of the new therapies are needed to be developed and undergo clinical trial.

References

1. Nelson RL. Epidemiology of fecal incontinence. Gastroenterology. 2004;126(1 Suppl 1):S3–7.
2. Ho YH, Muller R, Veitch C, Rane A, Durrheim D. Faecal incontinence: an unrecognised epidemic in rural North Queensland? Results of a hospital-based outpatient study. Aust J Rural Health. 2005;13:28–34.
3. Madoff RD, Williams JG, Caushaj PF. Fecal incontinence. N Engl J Med. 1992;326:1002–7.
4. Rao SS, American College of Gastroenterology Practice Parameters Committee. Diagnosis and management of fecal incontinence. American College of Gastroenterology Practice Parameters Committee. Am J Gastroenterol. 2004;99:1585–604.
5. Law PJ, Kamm MA, Bartram CI. Anal endosonography in the investigation of fecal incontinence. Br J Surg. 1991;78:312–4.
6. Woodfield CA, Krishnamoorthy S, Hampton BS, Brody JM. Imaging pelvic floor disorders: trend toward comprehensive MRI. AJR Am J Roentgenol. 2010;194:1640–9.
7. Barnett JL, Hasler WL, Camilleri M. American Gastroenterological Association medical position statement on anorectal testing techniques: American Gastroenterological Association. Gastroenterology. 1999;116:732–60.
8. Madoff RD, Parker SC, Varma MG, Lowry AC. Faecal incontinence in adults. Lancet. 2004;364:621–32.
9. Wald A. Fecal incontinence. Curr Treat Options Gastroenterol. 2005;8:319–24.
10. Read M, Read NW, Barber DC, Duthie HL. Effects of loperamide on anal sphincter function in patients complaining of chronic diarrhea with fecal incontinence and urgency. Dig Dis Sci. 1982;27:807–14.
11. Santoro GA, Eitan BZ, Pryde A, Bartolo DC. Open study of low-dose amitriptyline in the treatment of patients with idiopathic fecal incontinence. Dis Colon Rectum. 2000;43:1676–81.
12. MacLeod JH. Management of anal incontinence by biofeedback. Gastroenterology. 1987;93:291–4.
13. Ryn AK, Morren GL, Hallböök O, Sjödahl R. Long-term results of electromyographic biofeedback training for fecal incontinence. Dis Colon Rectum. 2000;43:1262–6.
14. Heymen S, Jones KR, Ringel Y, Scarlett Y, Whitehead WE. Biofeedback treatment of fecal incontinence: a critical review. Dis Colon Rectum. 2001;44:728–36.
15. Leroi AM, Dorival MP, Lecouturier MF, Saiter C, Welter ML, Touchais JY, Denis P. Pudendal neuropathy and severity of incontinence but not presence of an anal sphincter defect may determine the response to biofeedback therapy in fecal incontinence. Dis Colon Rectum. 1999;42:762–9.
16. Van Tets WF, Kuijpers JH, Bleijenberg G. Biofeedback treatment is ineffective in neurogenic fecal incontinence. Dis Colon Rectum. 1996;39:992–4.
17. Ratto C, Parello A, Donisi L, Litta F, De Simone V, Spazzafumo L, Giordano P. Novel bulking agent for faecal incontinence. Br J Surg. 2011;98(11):1644–52.
18. Luo C, Samaranayake CB, Plank LD, Bissett IP. Systematic review on the efficacy and safety of injectable bulking agents for passive faecal incontinence. Color Dis. 2010;12(4):296–303.
19. Altomare DF, La Torre F, Rinaldi M, Binda GA, Pescatori M. Carbon-coated microbeads anal injection in outpatient treatment of minor fecal incontinence. Dis Colon Rectum. 2008;51(4):432–5.
20. Kenefick NJ, Vaizey CJ, Malouf AJ, Norton CS, Marshall M, Kamm MA. Injectable silicone biomaterial for faecal incontinence due to internal anal sphincter dysfunction. Gut. 2002;51(2):225–8.
21. Felt-Bersma RJ. Temperature-controlled radiofrequency energy in patients with anal incontinence: an interim analysis of worldwide data. Gastroenterol Rep (Oxf). 2014;2(2):121–5.
22. Takahashi-Monroy T1, Morales M, Garcia-Osogobio S, Valdovinos MA, Belmonte C, Barreto C, Zarate X, Bada O, Velasco L. SECCA procedure for the treatment of fecal incontinence: results of five-year follow-up. Dis Colon Rectum. 2008;51(3):355–9.
23. Ruiz D, Pinto RA, Hull TL, Efron JE, Wexner SD. Does the radiofrequency procedure for fecal incontinence improve quality of life and incontinence at 1-year follow-up? Dis Colon Rectum. 2010;53(7):1041–6.
24. Vaizey CJ, Kamm MA, Nicholls RJ. Recent advances in the surgical treatment of faecal incontinence. Br J Surg. 1998;85:596–603.
25. Fang DT, Nivatvongs S, Vermeulen FD, Herman FN, Goldberg SM, Rothenberger DA. Overlapping sphincteroplasty for acquired anal incontinence. Dis Colon Rectum. 1984;27(11):720–2.
26. Young CJ, Mathur MN, Eyers AA, Solomon MJ. Successful overlapping anal sphincter repair. Dis Colon Rectum. 1998;41(3):344–9.
27. Halverson AL, Hull TL. Long-term outcome of overlapping anal sphincter repair. Dis Colon Rectum. 2002;45(3):345–8.
28. Malouf AJ, Norton CS, Engel AF, Nicholls RJ, Kamm MA. Long term results of overlapping anterior analsphincter repair for obstetric trauma. Lancet. 2000;355:260–5.
29. Baxter NN, Bravo Guttierez A, Lowry AC, Parker SC, Madoff RD. Long-term results of sphincteroplasty for acquired fecal incontinence (abstr). Dis Colon Rectum. 2003;45:A21–2.

30. Bravo Gutierrez A, Madoff RD, Lowry AC, Parker SC, Buie WD, Baxter NN. Long-term results of anterior sphincteroplasty. Dis Colon Rectum. 2004;47:727–32.
31. Madoff RD. Surgical treatment options for fecal incontinence. Gastroenterology. 2004;126:S48–54.
32. Leroi AM, Parc Y, Lehur PA, et al. Efficacy of sacral nerve stimulation for fecal incontinence: results of a multicenter double-blind crossover study. Ann Surg. 2005;242:662–9.
33. Tjandra JJ, Chan MK, Yeh CH, Murray-Green C. Sacral nerve stimulation is more effective than optimal medical therapy for severe fecal incontinence: a randomized, controlled study. Dis Colon Rectum. 2008;51:494–502.
34. Rosen HR, Urbarz C, Holzer B, Novi G, Schiessel R. Sacral nerve stimulation as a treatment for fecal incontinence. Gastroenterology. 2001;121:536–41.
35. Wong MT, Meurette G, Stangherlin P, Lehur PA. The magnetic anal sphincter versus the artificial bowel sphincter: a comparison of 2 treatments for fecal incontinence. Dis Colon Rectum. 2011;54:773–9.
36. Brouwer R, Duthie G. Sacral nerve neuromodulation is effective treatment for fecal incontinence in the presence of a sphincter defect, pudendal neuropathy, or previous sphincter repair. Dis Colon Rectum. 2010;53:273–8.
37. Hetzer FH. Fifteen years of sacral nerve stimulation: from an open procedure to a minimally invasive technique. Color Dis. 2011;13(Suppl 2):S1–4.
38. Matzel KE, Stadelmaier U, Hohenfellner M, Gall FP. Electrical stimulation of sacral spinal nerves for treatment of faecal incontinence. Lancet. 1995;346:1124–7.
39. Douglas JM, Smith LE. Recent concepts in fecal incontinence. Curr Womens Health Rep. 2001;1:67–71.
40. Spinelli M, Giardiello G, Arduini A, van den Hombergh U. New percutaneous technique of sacral nerve stimulation has high initial success rate: preliminary results. Eur Urol. 2003;43:70–4.

14 Pilonidal Disease

Jeong Eun Lee

14.1 Introduction

Pilonidal disease is a chronic inflammatory disease related to hair that occurs mainly in the gluteal cleft between the buttocks and can also occur in axilla or inguinal region. It has many controversial issues regarding its cause and treatment.

14.2 Etiology

In the past, it was considered that there is a congenital squamous epithelium in the midline of the gluteal cleft, which was the cause of inflammation. But in recent days, we are focusing on the idea that it is an acquired disease caused by foreign body reaction from hair. There are two hypotheses, one is that the ingrown hair induces foreign body reaction and the other is that the skin of the center buttocks is pulled due to the weight of buttocks which dilates hair follicles and becomes inflamed and spread to subcutaneous tissues, and the hair is secondarily invaded and becomes chronic [1]. It occurs mainly in men between 15 and 40 years of age. It shows asymptomatic small pit or simple cyst in the center of buttocks about 5 cm above the anus with pain and tenderness on pressure if it forms an abscess with cellulitis around the cyst. When it progresses to chronic phase, it shows various symptoms such as forming a purulent sinus (Fig. 14.1). And a sinus is formed in the central pit and sometimes has secondary branch from the formed inner tract [2].

14.3 Diagnosis

It is necessary to distinguish it from inflammatory diseases originating in the anus including anal fistula, hidradenitis suppurativa, and folliculitis through anal digital examination. Symptoms may vary from acute inflammation forming an abscess to a chronic exudate and painful sinus tract and can be easily diagnosed by physical

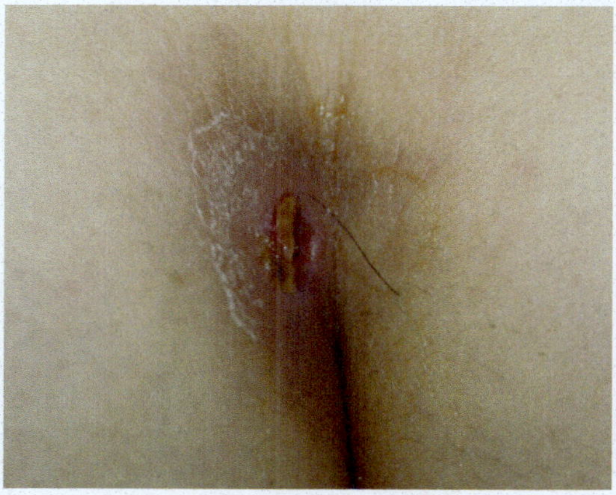

Fig. 14.1 A pilonidal sinus is a small hole or tunnel in the skin of the buttocks containing a hair

J. E. Lee (✉)
Colorectal Division, Department of Surgery, Hansol Hospital, Seoul, South Korea

D. K. Lee (ed.), *Practices of Anorectal Surgery*, https://doi.org/10.1007/978-981-13-1447-6_14

examination. If diagnosed with a pilonidal disease, special radiologic examination is not necessary, and X-ray and blood test are performed to measure the preoperative risk.

14.4 Treatment

Treatment for chronic pilonidal disease varies and is very controversial, but the principle of treatment is to completely remove the sinus tract, and recurrence has to be prevented after the excised skin is all healed.

14.4.1 Non-operative Treatment

Although the effect of antibiotics is limited, the use of combination of antibiotics may improve inflammation in patients with extensive cellulitis or in patients with impaired immune function or systemic disease [3, 4]. Because foreign body reaction is induced by ingrown hair inside the follicle and is the cause of pilonidal disease, laser treatment can be used as a primary treatment or adjuvant treatment [5–7]. Prior to phenol (1–2 ml of 80% phenol solution) or fibrin glue injection, all hair and debris must be removed and curetted from the sinus. Phenol is injected to remove granulation tissue and promote healing process, and patients should be hospitalized with proper pain control because the injection may cause severe pain. Incidentally discovered asymptomatic pilonidal sinus does not require prophylactic surgery.

14.4.2 Operative Treatment

14.4.2.1 Incision and Drainage

Most of the patients who visited clinic with pain showed abscess or cellulitis. It is common in patients that cellulitis is accompanied by an abscess in subcutaneous fat layer. Abscess can be treated by simple incision and drainage in about 60% without additional surgery, but in 10–15%, it recurred [8, 9]. When incision and drainage are performed, curettage is not necessary. In acute phase, excision of midline pits with incision and drainage does not help in healing or in recurrence.

14.4.2.2 Wide Excision and Primary Closure or Marsupialization

The principle of pilonidal disease surgery is wide excision to completely remove all inflammatory tissue and pilonidal cyst and purulent sinus. Anatomically in sacrococcygeal area, there is not enough skin, and subcutaneous layer is thin; therefore, wound healing is often difficult after suture of the wide excision. In case of incomplete wide excision, there can be high recurrence; there have been various surgical methods introduced to reduce recurrence and complications which occur in the wound healing process. In our hospital, we mainly use wide excision and open or marsupialization method. Patients are prepared with NPO from midnight prior to the surgery but no need for mechanical bowel preparation. It is mainly performed in prone jackknife position under spinal anesthesia (Fig. 14.2).

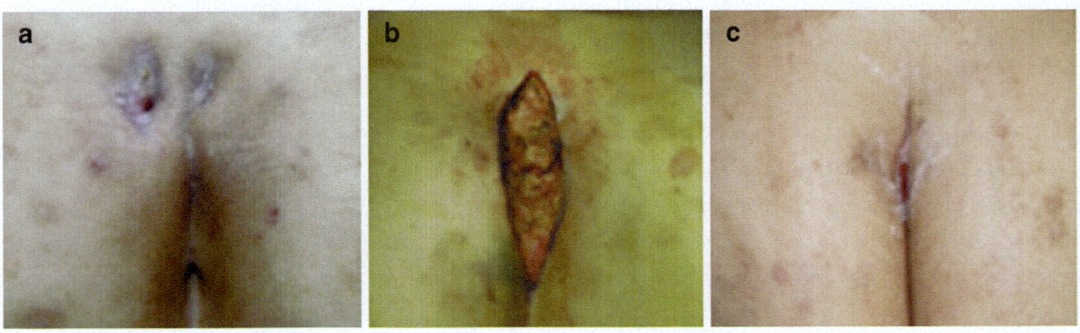

Fig. 14.2 Before and after surgical excision for pilonidal disease. (**a**) Showing midline pit with sinus tract before operation. (**b**) Immediately after operation with wide excision and lay open. (**c**) Four weeks later following operation showing nearly epithelized wounds

Stage 1 Attach tape to both sides of sacrococcygeal area to have better vision and avoid pulling too much. Check openings pits, and make sure there is no secondary tract. Methylene blue can be used to identify the excision range as it can be stained to a part of normal tissue; do not apply excessive pressure at injection, and be cautious not to excise too much the tissue. Use marking pen to design the excision area.

Stage 2 The skin including the opening pits is excised in an elliptical shape and dissected until the fascia appears, and the entire superior subcutaneous tissue is excised. The remained inflammatory tissue can be the cause of recurrence, so they should be completely removed.

Stage 3 After wide excision, the wound is checked for hemostasis and cleaned with dilute betadine solution. And suture the wound using an absorbable suture like 2-0 or 3-0 Vicryl. If the wound is not pulled sufficiently, marsupialization is performed with an absorbable suture to the edge of the wound, and wet dressing is performed.

After the surgery, the patients should lay down in a prone position or a lateral decubitus position, and normal dietary can be taken after 6 hours. Prior to the surgery, second-generation cephalosporin antibiotics are administered intravenously, and postoperative antibiotics are administered orally for 3 days after the surgery. Half of the stitches are removed at first week after the surgery, and the rest are removed at second week after the surgery. In the case of wet dressing with an open wound, for 5 days after the surgery, change dressing daily and then shower gently and dry. Hematoma from postoperative bleeding can be the cause of infection or wound disruption; therefore, intensive hemostasis is essential, and if possible, do not use drain tube to prevent infection. In open wound, healing usually takes more than 2 months and recurrence rate varies from 0 to 30% [10]. As a re-ingrowing hair into the natal cleft is the cause of recurrence of inflammation, it would be helpful to remove the hairs on the buttocks with an electric shaver once every 2–3 weeks to reduce recurrence rate. There is a report that marsupialization accelerates healing of the wound [11, 12].

14.4.2.3 Bascom's Operation

In 1965 few doctors insisted on incising only the central pit area after removing the hair and drainage as pilonidal disease is from foreign body reaction by ingrown hair which made sinus [13]. Bascom's extended theory is that the inflammation from hair follicles is the main cause of sinus tract and should be removed. Therefore, the treatment varies to the degree and condition of inflammation. All surgeries were performed under local anesthesia in outpatient clinic. In the case of chronic inflammation, hair follicles should be incised under the midline including only the minimum healthy tissue leaving 2–4 mm diameter of the wound. In addition, leaving about one knuckle from the midline, incise vertically into the center, and curette any hair or granulation tissue using gauze. Excise any sinus tract and lateral incision is left without suture [10]. Postoperative recurrence rate is about 10–15%, but in the case of recurrence, 80% were cured with this surgical method [10, 14, 15].

14.4.2.4 Advancement Fap

Advantage of advancement flap is that after removing all sinus tract and infected subcutaneous tissue, using the surrounding healthy tissue, it can be sutured immediately without tension. Also, with wide excision, recurrence rate is relatively low. Z-plasty [16], V-Y advancement flap [17, 18], rhomboid flap [19], and gluteus maximus myocutaneous flap [20] are used and classified by shape. As of complications, there can be hematoma, infection, or abscess under the flap. In these flap procedures, the time to wound healing is reduced by 2–3 weeks, and recurrence rate varies from 4% to 38% [20, 21].

In the case of recurrent pilonidal disease, pathophysiologic process is similar to that of the primary disease; treatment depends on acute or chronic phase, size of lesion, and previous operation method. If chronic recurrent pilonidal disease is left untreated, squamous cell carcinoma can be developed in about 0.1%. For the treatment of carcinoma, wide excision with additional chemotherapy and radiation therapy can be performed, but the prognosis is poor [22].

14.5 Summary

Pilonidal disease is a chronic inflammatory disease related to hair that occurs mainly in the gluteal cleft between the buttocks and can also occur in axilla or inguinal region. It has many controversial issues regarding its cause and treatment including wide excision and primary closure or left open wound.

References

1. Karydakis GE. The etiology of pilonidal sinus. Hellenic Arm Forc Med Rev. 1975;7:411–6.
2. Hull TL, Wu J. Pilonidal disease. Surg Clin N Am. 2002;82:1169–85.
3. Hanley PH. Acute pilonidal abscess. Surg Gynecol Obstet. 1980;150:9–11.
4. Nelson J, Billingham R. Pilonidal disease and hidradenitis suppurativa. In: Wolff BG, Fleshman JW, Beck DE, et al., editors. The ASCRS textbook of colon and rectal surgery. New York: Springer; 2007. p. 228–35.
5. Lukish JR, Kindelan T, Marmon LM, et al. Laser epilation is a safe and effective therapy for teenagers with pilonidal disease. J Pediatr Surg. 2009;44:28205.
6. Conroy FJ, Kandamany N, Mahaffey PJ. Laser depilation and hygiene: preventing recurrent pilonidal sinus disease. J Plast Reconstr Aesthet Surg. 2008;61:1069–72.
7. Schulze SM, Patel N, Hertzog D, et al. Treatment of pilonidal disease with laser epilation. Am Surg. 2006;72:534–7.
8. Jensen SL, Harling H. Prognosis after simple incision and dreainage for a first-episode acute pilonidal abscess. Br J Surg. 1988;75:60–1.
9. Webb PM, Wysocki AP. Does pilonidal abscess heal quicker with off-midline incision and drainage ? Tech Coloproctol. 2011;15:179–83.
10. Bascom J. Pilonidal disease: origin from follicles of hairs and results of follicle removal as treatment. Surgery. 1980;87(5):567–72.
11. Oncel M, Kurt N, Kement M, et al. Excision and marsupialization versus sinus excision for the treatment of limited chronic pilonidal disease; a prospective randomized trial. Tech Coloproctol. 2002;6:165.
12. Al-Hassan HK, Francis IM, Neglen P. Primary closure or secondary granulation after excision of pilonidal sinus? Acta Chir Scand. 1990;156:695–9.
13. Lord PH, Millar DM. Pilonidal sinus: a simple treatment. Br J Surg. 1965;52:298–300.
14. Mosquera DA, Quayle JB. Bascom's operation for pilonidal sinus. J R Soc Med. 1995;88(1):45–6.
15. Senapati A, Cripps NP, Thompson MR. Bascom's operation in the day-surgical management of symptomatic pilonidal sinus. Br J Surg. 2000;87(8):1067–70.
16. Mansoory A, Dickson D. Z-plasty for treatment of disease of the pilonidal sinus. Surg Gynecol Obstet. 1982;155(3):409–11.
17. Schoeller T, Wechselberger G, Otto A, Papp C. Definite surgical treatment of complicated recurrent pilonidal disease with a modified fasciocutaneous V-Y advancement flap. Surgery. 1997;121(3):258–63.
18. Dýlek ON, Bekereciodlu M. Role of simple V-Y advancement flap in the treatment of complicated pilonidal sinus. Eur J Surg. 1998;164(12):961–4.
19. Milito G, Cortese F, Casciani CU. Rhomboid flap procedure for pilonidal sinus: results from 67 cases. Int J Color Dis. 1998;13(3):113–5.
20. Rosen W, Davidson JS. Gluteus maximus musculocutaneous flap for the treatment of recalcitrant pilonidal disease. Ann Plast Surg. 1996;37:293–7.
21. Solla JA, Rothenberger DA. Chronic pilonidal disease. An assessment of 150 cases. Dis Colon Rectum. 1990;33:758–61.
22. de Bree E, Zoetmulder FAN, Christodoulakis M, et al. Treatment of malignancy arising in pilonidal disease. Ann Surg Oncol. 2001;8:60–4.

15 Hidradenitis Suppurativa

Jeong Eun Lee

15.1 Introduction

Hidradenitis suppurativa is a chronic recurrent inflammation of the apocrine sweat gland, but to be accurate, it begins at the follicular portion of the folliculopilosebaceous unit. It occurs most commonly in the axilla and can also occur in the buttocks, perineum, inguinal area, and breast [1] (Fig. 15.1). The exact cause is unclear, but when follicular unit is blocked and dilated by remained keratin, inflammation occurs and spreads to the surrounding area caused by rupture and forms abscess or sinus. Then secondary tract appears, and the lesion gradually extends into dermal layer and subcutaneous tissue. If the treatment is not performed in time, it becomes chronic and scars appear with wrinkle which deteriorates the quality of life. When inflammation occurs, it is located deeper in the skin compared to the other general abscess and spreads transversely along the subcutaneous fat layer, and it does not respond well to antibiotic treatment [2].

Multiple inflammatory lesion and scars involving entire gluteal and perianal area.

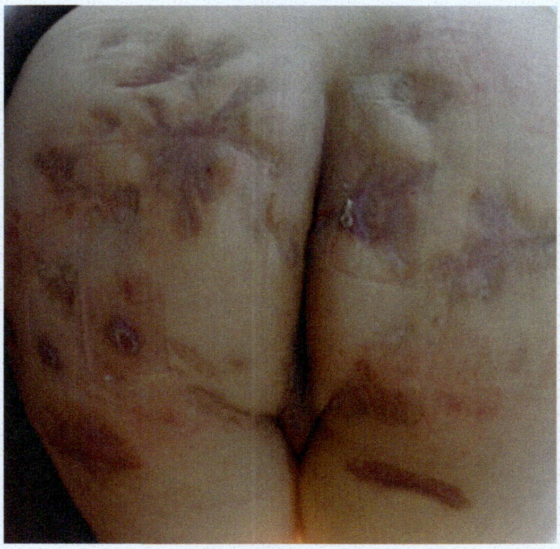

Fig. 15.1 Hidradenitis suppurativa

15.2 Etiology

The cause of hidradenitis suppurativa is considered to be the sweat gland or follicular occlusion, but their underlying cause is not clear. It is commonly found in young patients between the age of 16 and 40, and more common in women, but more common in men in perianal and genital area [3]. A third of patients have family history, and the causative factors are known to be obesity, acne, filthy hygiene, and hyperhidrosis, and it is reported to have relation with smoking or endocrine abnormalities such as excessive androgen, progesterone depletion [4]. In women, symptoms

J. E. Lee (✉)
Colorectal Division, Department of Surgery, Hansol Hospital, Seoul, South Korea
e-mail: cybexgirl@hanmail.net

D. K. Lee (ed.), *Practices of Anorectal Surgery*, https://doi.org/10.1007/978-981-13-1447-6_15

improve after menopause, but in men, it can continue to progress with age [5–7].

15.3 Diagnosis

It can be easily diagnosed by combining type, recurrence, chronicity, and location of inflammation. It is necessary to distinguish it from other infectious anal diseases such as anal fistula, Crohn's disease, tuberculosis, pilonidal disease, and infected sebaceous cyst through physical examination. If hidradenitis suppurativa is left neglected for long period, it can cause complications such as anemia, hypoproteinemia, and fistula formation to surrounding pelvic organs, and although rare, it can also occur squamous cell carcinoma [2, 8, 9]. There is a report on the association with Crohn's disease, and sometimes it is difficult to distinguish them and biopsies should be done through colonoscopy after basic blood tests as needed. If Crohn's disease is mistaken for hidradenitis suppurativa and excision is performed, unhealed wounds can be left that can be difficult to heal [10, 11].

In assessing the extent of disease, Hurley classifications is used more often clinically [12].

15.3.1 Hurley Staging

- Stage I: Abscess formation, single or multiple, without sinus tracts and cicatrization
- Stage II: Recurrent abscesses with tract formation and cicatrization, single or multiple, widely separated lesions
- Stage III: Diffuse or near-diffuse involvement, or multiple interconnected tracts and abscesses across the entire area

Stage I is most common (68%), and stage II is about 28%, and stage III is within 5% [13].

15.4 Treatment

Hidradenitis suppurativa has various symptoms and does not have single therapy for complete cure. In the early stage, conservative treatment can reduce pain and improve uncomfortable symptoms. Clean skin hygiene is essential, and hands should be washed, and avoid using irritant material which can cause wound. Ultimately, surgical treatment is required in the case of severe inflammation or repeated symptoms.

15.4.1 Medical Treatment

Medical treatment includes antibiotic therapy, hormonal treatment, and immunosuppressive agents. In acute phase, the target is to eliminate the uncomfortable symptom including pain. Keep affected area clean and avoid dairy products, and reduce sugar content to reduce weight. In antibiotic treatment, mainly the oral antibiotics such as cephalosporin, erythromycin, and tetracycline are used, which are effective against *Staphylococcus*, *Streptococcus*, and *Escherichia coli*. Topical antimicrobial agents such as hexachlorophene, povidone iodine, and topical clindamycin are also used [14, 15]. However, long-term use of antibiotics does not help in prevention and treatment of hidradenitis suppurativa [16]. But symptoms improve with the use of isotretinoin (13-cis-retinoic acid), an acne treatment drug or steroids, and androgen agent reduces the production of androgen [17–19]. Also immunosuppressive agents such as cyclosporine and radiation therapy were somewhat effective, but there is no report on the definite effect; therefore, side effects due to immunosuppression should be considered with the treatment [20, 21]. TNF-alpha inhibitors and adalimumab are also reported to be effective in the treatment of hidradenitis suppurativa.

15.4.2 Operative Treatment

Chronic, recurrent, and severe hidradenitis suppurativa requires surgical treatment. There is much controversy about surgical methods, and surgical procedures vary depending on the location, extent, and chronicity of the lesion [22].

15.4.2.1 Simple Incision and Drainage or Unroofing

It is effective in rapid relief of symptoms in acute phase, but in most cases, they recurred within 3 months. This procedure should be performed with severe pain and necessary for additional surgery after inflammation has subsided to some extent [23].

15.4.2.2 Unroofing of Sinus Tracts and Marsupialization

Using probe, incise along the tract and widen to remove granulation tissue by tract curettage and expect secondary healing [6]. Marsupialize the edge of wound for fast healing. If the affected area is wide, it can be useful, but recurrent rate is high and needs sufficient postoperative wound management [24, 25].

15.4.2.3 Limited Local Excision or Wide Excision

For small lesion it can be performed under local anesthesia, but for wide excision, it should be performed in prone jackknife position under spinal anesthesia. For small lesion, it can be sutured after local excision, and the patient's satisfaction is high, but it has high risk of infection [26]. For wide excision, if excision includes normal fat tissue under the tract, wound healing may take longer time; therefore, incise and excise inflammatory area along the tract, and then curette granulation tissue leaving epithelium of the base [27]. Attempts to cover the excised wound with skin graft or flaps have high risk of infection [28]. After surgery, the wound should be wet dressed with dilute betadine solution every day. Wound complications like bleeding and infection can occur and take longer to heal [14]. Recurrence after wide excision should not be taken as treatment failure but as characteristic of the disease [29, 30].

15.5 Recurrence

In incision and drainage, immediate pain relief can be obtained, but in most cases, it recurs and requires additional surgery. Recurrence rate of wide excision has been reported to vary from 17% to 67%; as the reports vary in extent of inflammation and duration of disease, it is difficult to have accurate comparison [6, 31–33]. Mehdizadeh and others reported that wide excision (13%) had less recurrence than local excision (22%) or unroofing (27%) [34]. Recurrence was reported higher with wider inflammation and in more scattered lesion and with primary suture [35].

15.6 Summary

Hidradenitis suppurativa is a chronic recurrent inflammation of the apocrine sweat gland, but to be accurate, it begins at the follicular portion of the folliculopilosebaceous unit. It occurs most commonly in the axilla and can also occur in the buttocks, perineum, inguinal area, and breast. Hidradenitis suppurativa has various symptoms and does not have single therapy for complete cure. Chronic, recurrent, and severe hidradenitis suppurativa requires surgical treatment.

References

1. Patil S, Apurwa A, Nadkarni N, Agarwal S, Chaudhari P, Gautam M. Hidradenitis Suppurativa: inside and out. Indian J Dermatol. 2018;63(2):91–8.
2. Mitchell KM, Beck DE. Hidradenitis suppurativa. Surg Clin North Am. 2002;82:1187–97.
3. Brown TJ, Rosen T, Orengo IF. Hidradenitis supurativa. South Med J. 1998;91:1107–14.
4. König A, Lehmann C, Rompel R, Happle R. Cigarette smoking as a triggering factor of hidradenitis suppurativa. Dermatology. 1999;198(3):261–4.
5. Mortimer PS, Dawber R{, Gales MA, et al. Medication of hidradenitis suppurativa by androgens. Br Med J 1986;292:245–248.
6. Wiltz O, Scoetz DJ, Murray JJ, et al. Perianal hidradenitis suppurativa. The lahey Clinic Experience. Dis Colon Rectum. 1990;33:731–4.
7. Stellon AJ, Wakeling M. Hidradenitis suppurativa associated with use of oral contraceptives. BMJ. 1989;298(6665):28–9.
8. Perez-Diaz D, Calvo-Serrano M, Martinez-Hijosa E, et al. Squamous cell carcinoma complicating perianal hidradenitis suppurativa. Int J Color Dis. 1995;10:225–8.
9. Pérez-Diaz D, Calvo-Serrano M, Mártinez-Hijosa E, Fuenmayor-Valera L, Muñoz-Jiménez F, Turégano-Fuentes F, Del Valle E. Squamous cell car-

cinoma complicating perianal hidradenitis suppurativa. Int J Color Dis. 1995;10(4):225–8.
10. Burrows NP, Jones RR. Crohn's disease in association with hidradenitis suppurativa. Br J Dermatol. 1992;126(5):523.
11. Gower-Rousseau C, Maunoury V, Colombel JF, Coulom P, Piette F, Cortot A, Paris JC. Hidradenitis suppurativa and Crohn's disease in two families: a significant association? Am J Gastroenterol. 1992;87(7):928.
12. Hurley H. Axillary hyperhidrosis, apocrine bromhidrosis, hidradenitis suppurativa, and familial benign pemphigus: surgical approach. In: Roenigh RRH, editor. Dermatologic surgery. New York: Marcel Dekker; 1989. p. 729–39.
13. Canoui-Poitrine F, Revuz JE, Wolkenstein P, et al. Clinical characteristics of a series of 302 French patients with hidradenitis suppurativa, with an analysis of factors associated with disease severity. J Am Acad Dermatol. 2009;61:51–7.
14. Thornton JP, Abcarian H. Surgical treatment of perianal and perineal hidradenitis suppurativa. Dis Colon Rectum. 1978;21:573–7.
15. Clemmensen OJ. Topical treatment of hidradenitis suppurativa with clindamycin. Int J Dermatol. 1983;22(5):325–8.
16. Culp CE. Chronic hidradenitis suppurativa of the anal canal. A surgical skin disease. Dis Colon Rectum. 1983;26(10):669–76.
17. Rubin RJ, Chinn BT. Perianal hidradenitis suppurativa. Surg Clin North Am. 1994;74:1317–25.
18. Brown CF, Gallup DG, Brown VM. Hidradenitis suppurativa of the anogenital region: response to isotretinoin. Am J Obstet Gynecol. 1988;158(1):12–5.
19. Hogan DJ, Light MJ. Successful treatment of hidradenitis suppurativa with acitretin. J Am Acad Dermatol. 1988;19(2. Pt 1):355–6.
20. Sawers RS, Randall VA, Ebling FS. Control of hidradenitis suppurativa in women using combined antiandrogen(ciproterone acetate) and oestrogen therapy. Br J Dermatol. 1986;115:269–74.
21. Gupta AK, Ellis CN, Cooper KD, Nickoloff BJ, Ho VC, Chan LS, Hamilton TA, Tellner DC, Griffiths CE, Voorhees JJ. Oral cyclosporine for the treatment of alopecia areata. A clinical and immunohistochemical analysis. J Am Acad Dermatol. 1990;22:242–50.
22. Janse I, Bieniek A, Horváth B, Matusiak Ł. Surgical procedures in hidradenitis suppurativa. Dermatol Clin. 2016;34(1):97–109.
23. Mehdizadeh A, Hazen PG, Bechara FG, Zwingerman N, Moazenzadeh M, Bashash M, Sibbald RG, Alavi A. Recurrence of hidradenitis suppurativa after surgical management: a systematic review and meta-analysis. J Am Acad Dermatol. 2015;73(5 Suppl 1):S70–7.
24. Kohorst JJ, Baum CL, Otley CC, Roenigk RK, Schenck LA, Pemberton JH, Dozois EJ, Tran NV, Senchenkov A, Davis MD. Surgical management of hidradenitis suppurativa: outcomes of 590 consecutive patients. Dermatol Surg. 2016;42(9):1030–40.
25. Danby FW. Commentary: unroofing for hidradenitis suppurativa, why and how. J Am Acad Dermatol. 2010;63(3):481.e1–3.
26. van Rappard DC, Mooij JE, Mekkes JR. Mild to moderate hidradenitis suppurativa treated with local excision and primary closure. J Eur Acad Dermatol Venereol. 2012;26(7):898–902.
27. Brown SC, Kazzazi N, Lord PH. Surgical treatment of perineal hidradenitis suppurativa with special reference to recognition of the perianal form. Br J Surg. 1986;73:987–0.
28. Rompel R, Petres J. Long-term results of wide surgical excision in 106 patients with hidradenitis suppurativa. Dermatol Surg. 2000;26(7):638–43.
29. Burney RE. 35-year experience with surgical treatment of hidradenitis suppurativa. World J Surg. 2017;41(11):2723–30.
30. Posch C, Monshi B, Quint T, Vujic I, Lilgenau N, Rappersberger K. The role of wide local excision for the treatment of severe hidradenitis suppurativa (Hurley grade III): retrospective analysis of 74 patients. J Am Acad Dermatol. 2017;77(1):123–9.
31. Menderes A, Sunay O, Vayvada H, Yilmaz M. Surgical management of hidradenitis suppurativa. Int J Med Sci. 2010;7(4):240.
32. Banerjee AK. Surgical treatment of hidradenitis suppurativa. Br J Surg. 1992;79:863–6.
33. Wilta O, Schoetz KJ Jr, Murray JJ, Roberts PL, Coller JA, Weidenheimer MC. Perianal hidradenitis suppurativa. The Lahey Clinic experience. Dis Colon Rectum. 1990;33:73–4.
34. Mehdizadeh A, Jazen PG, Bechara FG, et al. Recurrence of hidradenitis suppurativa after surgical management a systematic review and meta-analysis. J Am Acad Dermatol. 2015;73(5.)(Suppl):S70–7.
35. Watson JD. Hidradenitis suppurativa-a clinical review. Br J Plast Surg. 1985;38:567–9.

16 Condyloma Accuminatum

Sanghwa Yu

16.1 Introduction

Condyloma is the most common disease of sexually transmitted diseases (STDs) of anorectal region coming from human papillomavirus (HPV) infection. There are more than 40 HPV types that infect genitourinary tract and anal region. HPVs are divided into two subtypes – the high-risk HPV subtype (HPV-16, HPV-18, HPV-33, HPV-53, HPV-56, HPV-58, HPV-61) and the low-risk HPV subtype – based on malignant and association, and the majority (90%) of anal warts are caused by low-risk HPV subtypes 6 and 11 [1–3]. They are known to be transmitted by sexual intercourse (especially anal sex), but in clinic, there are cases frequently observed that are not associated with sexual intercourse. Condyloma near genitalia are highly contagious, about 50% can be infected by only single sexual contact, and in most cases, the skin lesion appears 2~3 months after sexual intercourse.

In most cases, development appears after 6–10 months of latent period, but some cases remain subclinical for several years which make it difficult to determine exact route of infection. On the other hand, most HPV infections are reported to be resolved within 1–2 years by one's immune system, and about 90% of the infection is completely cured after 5 years [4, 5].

Warts' shape lesion occurs in either solitary or multiple around perianal skin and in anal canal (Fig. 16.1). In initial stage, it starts with shiny small papule, but as time passes, the papules gather and form berry or comb shape (Fig. 16.2).

These papillary shape tissues are weak and easy to be ulcerated, accompanied by discharge; it sometimes associates bleeding due to common anal pruritus.

It can be easily diagnosed visually or with anoscopy in the perianal skin and anal canal. Biopsy is performed when condyloma is in atypical condition such as pigmented or indurated, affixed to underlying tissue, or accompanied by bleeding or ulceration with intraepithelial or infiltrative squamous cell carcinoma (Fig. 16.3).

16.2 Treatment

Patients should be instructed not to have sexual activities during treatment due to risk of transmission of infection or reinfection, and if possible, the partner should be advised to have examination and treated together. Treatment is focused on removing warts locally rather than treatment for infection. Several factors should be considered prior to choosing the treatment, such as the location and degree of warts and preference of the patients.

S. Yu (✉)
Colorectal Division, Department of Surgery, Hansol Hospital, Seoul, South Korea
e-mail: ysh@hansolh.co.kr

D. K. Lee (ed.), *Practices of Anorectal Surgery*, https://doi.org/10.1007/978-981-13-1447-6_16

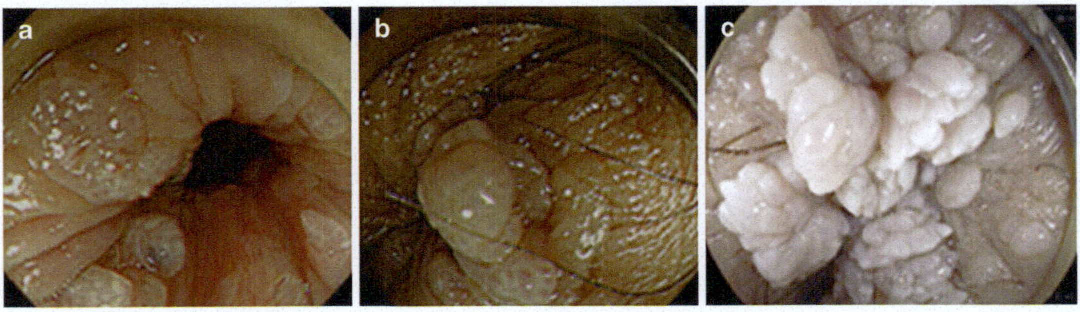

Fig. 16.1 Warts shape lesion. (**a**) Solitary wart around the perianal skin. (**b**) Multiple warts around perianal skin. (**c**) Multiple warts around perianal skin and internal anal canal

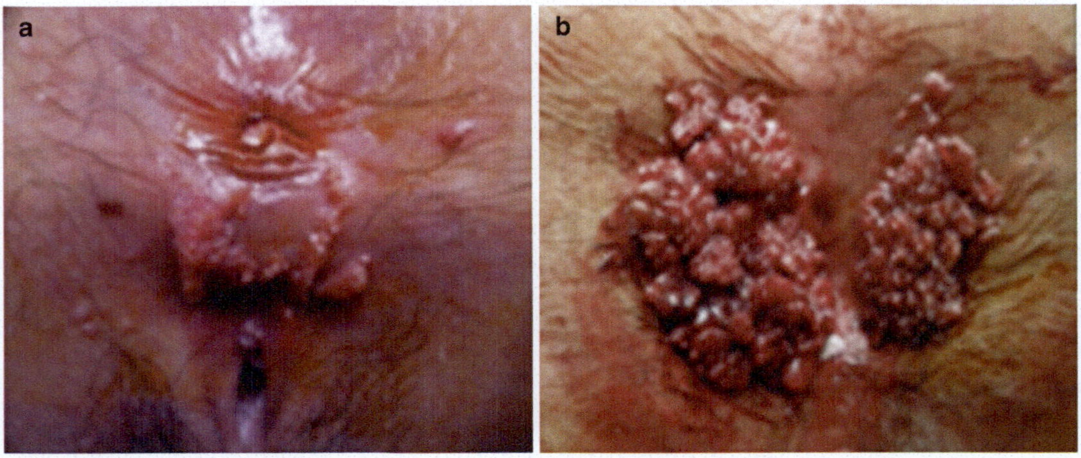

Fig. 16.2 Various condyloma shapes. (**a**) In early stage, small papule around perianal skin. (**b**) As time passes, papules gather and form berry or comb shape

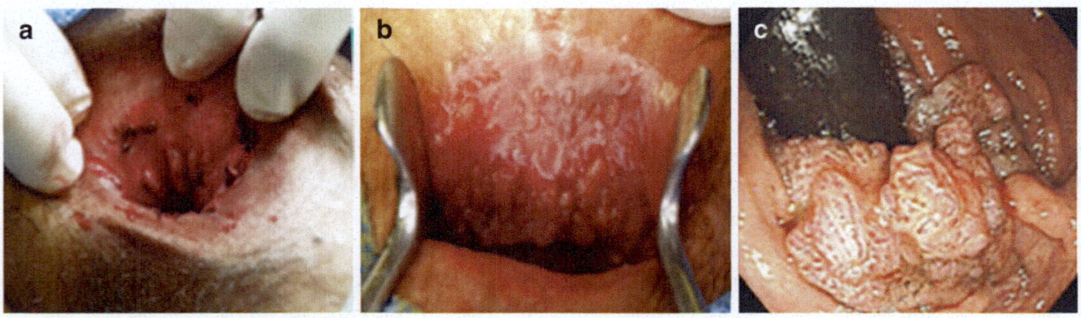

Fig. 16.3 Atypical condyloma. (**a**) Condyloma with pigmentation. (**b**) Condyloma with induration affixed to underlying tissue. (**c**) Accompanied by bleeding or ulcerated with intraepithelial or infiltrative squamous cell carcinoma

16.2.1 Medical Treatment

16.2.1.1 Imiquimod Cream (Aldara®)

Since 2010, imiquimod cream has been approved by the Food and Drug Administration (FDA) for the treatment of external warts in the patients aged over 12 years. Imiquimod is a potent immunomodulator and stimulates immune system to heal lesions. The use is limited as the safety and efficacy have not been evaluated in pregnant, breastfeeding, or immunosuppressed patients or in the patients with condyloma intravaginal, cervical, rectal, or anal canal. Pruritus, a burning sensation, pain, or skin ulcers are the side effects, and some patients complain of systemic side effects such as headache, myalgia, or weakness. Because of these systemic side effects, 3.75% cream has been clinically used, but comparing healing rate with the 5% cream, it is comparably low (56% vs. 36.6%), and recurrence rate is low as 13% in the 5% cream [6, 7].

16.2.1.2 High-Dose Cimetidine

High-dose cimetidine has an immunomodulatory effect. It inhibits function via H2-receptor on suppressor T cell and stimulates activation of natural killer (NK) cells and helper T cell which are cell-mediated immunity and is known to destroy virus [8, 9].

Treatment is to be effective from 80% of the patients with dosed 6–8 weeks with 2–3 times a day and 25 to 40 mg/kg. But this treatment is reported as not effective in the13 study of adult patients; therefore, high-dose cimetidine could be considered to be used with other standard therapies for warts in children.

16.2.1.3 Podophyllotoxin

Podophyllotoxin inhibits cell division and causes necrosis of condyloma within 2 days. 0.15% cream or podophyllotoxin jell should be used two times a day for 3 days, and then give it a resting period for 4 days, and this treatment can be used up to 4 weeks. In some patients, there are local side effects like pruritic, stinging, or burning of skin trouble. Success rate is 62.2% and recurrence rate is 55% [6, 10].

16.2.1.4 Sinecatechins (Polyphenon E)

Sinecatechins is a botanical medication first to be approved by FDA. It is not yet clearly announced of its action mechanism, but it is considered to be treating condyloma by inhibiting cell development and accelerating discharge of cytokine. Use 15% sinecatechins cream for 4 months, three times a week, and the results show similar to the other local application with cure rate of 54.9% and recurrence rate of 6.5%. And it is reported to be rare for local side effects like burning skin trouble [11].

16.2.1.5 Trichloroacetic Acid (TCA)

Trichloroacetic acid is a strong corrosive chemical which cauterizes condyloma. Careful not to apply on healthy skin tissue around the lesion, and it is not recommended to use as treatment on condyloma in anal canal. Cure rate is fairly high as 70–81%, but also the recurrence rate is as high as 36% [12].

16.2.2 Surgical Treatment

Surgical excision is the oldest treatment for condyloma and is the most effective treatment with cure rate of 94%. Also, it can both be applied to perianal condyloma and also condyloma in intravaginal, cervical, rectal, or anal canal. Electric excision can be combined for small lesion as it is easy to use; however, it leaves scars and high recurrence rate.

16.3 Prevention

As of now, there is no ideal treatment for condyloma; therefore, prevention is best treatment. FDA-approved Gardasil as vaccination in 2006 as first 4vHPV (HPV 6, 11, 16, 18) for girls and women aged 9–29 with condyloma [13, 14]. In many studies, it is reported that seroconversion rate is over 97.5% through vaccination, and this rate is much higher than seroconversion rate of one's self immune system (54–67%); therefore, vaccination is recommended for effective condyloma prevention [15].

16.4 Summary

Condyloma is the most common disease of sexually transmitted diseases (STDs) of anorectal region coming from human papillomavirus (HPV) infection. Treatment is focused on removing warts locally rather than treatment for infection. Several factors should be considered prior to choosing the treatment.

References

1. Human papilloma viruses. In: IARC monographs on the evaluation of carcinogenic risks to human, vol. 90. Lyon: International Agency for Research on Cancer; 2007. p. 209–22.
2. Anic GM, Lee JH, Stockwell H, et al. Incidence and human papillomavirus (HPV) type distribution genital warts in a multinational cohort of men: the HPV in men study. J Infect Dis. 2011;204:1886–92.
3. Sturegard E, Johansson H, Ekstrom J, Hasson BG, Johnsson A, Gustafsson E, Dillner J, Forslund O. Human papillomavirus typing in reporting condyloma. Sex Transm Dis. 2013;40:123–9.
4. Elfgren K, Kalantari M, Moberger B, Hagmar B, Dillner J. A population-based five-year follow-up study of cervical human papillomavirus infection. Am J Obstet Gynecol. 2000;183:561–7.
5. Massad LS, Xie X, Darragh T, et al. Genital warts and vulvar intraepithelial neoplasia: natural history and effects of treatment and human immunodeficiency virus infection. Obstet Gynecol. 2011;118:831–9.
6. Edwards A, Atma-Ram A, Thin RN. Podophyllotoxin 0.5% v. podophyllin 20% to treat penile warts. Genitourin Med. 1988;64:263–5.
7. Chuang Chi-Mu, Monie A, Hung Chien-fu, Wu T-C. Treatment with Imiquimod enhances antitumor immunity induced by therapeutic HPV DNA vaccination. J Biomed Sci. 2010;17:31–40.
8. Chang Ook Park, Kee Yang Chung, Woo Gil Chung. Treatment of verruca plana with high dose cimetidine therapy. Korean J Dermatol. 2005;43(4):475–9.
9. Dasher DA, Burkhart CN, Morrell DS. Immunotherapy for childhood warts. Pediatr Ann. 2009;38(7):373–9.
10. Lacey CJN, Goodall RL, Rangarson Tennvall G, Maw R, Kinghorn GR, Fisk PG, Barton S, Byren I. Randomised controlled trial and economic evaluation of podophyllotoxin solution, podophyllotoxin cream, and podophyllin in the treatment of genital warts. Sex Transm Infect. 2003;79:270–5.
11. Tatti S, Stockfleth E, Beutner KR, Tawfik K, Elsasser U, Weyrauch P, Mescheder A. Polyphenon E: a new treatment for external anogenital warts. Br J Dermatol. 2010;162:176–84.
12. Abdullah AN, Walzman M, Wade A. Treatment of external genital warts comparing cryotherapy (liquid nitrogen) and trichloroacetic acid. Sex Transm Dis. 1993;20:344–5.
13. Markowitz LE, Dunne EF, Saraiy M, et al. Human papillomavirus vaccination: recommendation of the Advisory Committee on Immunization Practices. MMWR Morb Mortal Wkly Rep. 2014;63(RR-05):1–30.
14. Petrosky E, Bocchini JA Jr, Hariri S, et al. Use of 9-valent human papillomavirus (HPV) vaccine: updated HPV vaccination recommendations of the Advisory Committee on Immunization Practices. MMWR Morb Mortal Wkly Rep. 2015;64:300–4.
15. Block SL, Nolan T, Sattler C, Barr E, Giacoletti KE, Marchant CD, Castellsagué X, Rusche SA, Lukac S, Bryan JT, Cavanaugh PF Jr, Reisinger KS. Protocol 016 Study Group.: Comparison of immunogenicity and reactogenicity of a prophylactic quadrivalent human papillomavirus (types 6,11,16 and 18) L1 virus-like particle vaccine in male and female adolescents and young adult women. Pediatrics. 2006;118:2135–45.

The manufacturer's authorised representative in the EU is Springer Nature Customer Service Centre GmbH, Europaplatz 3, 69115 Heidelberg, Germany. If you have any concerns regarding our products, please contact ProductSafety@springernature.com

Printed and bound by CPI Group (UK) Ltd, Croydon, CR0 4YY
25/09/2026
02222841-0020